Intermittent Fasting For Women Over 50

The 21 Day Guide for Fast and Easy Weight Loss, Burn Fat and Slow Aging through Metabolic Process of Autopaghy, Increase Energy and Improve Your Life Quality

Dr. Jason Stephens

publisher for any reparation, damages, or monetary loss due to the information herein, either directly or indirectly.

Respective authors own all copyrights not held by the publisher.

The information herein is offered for informational purposes solely, and is universal as so. The presentation of the information is without contract or any type of guarantee assurance.

The trademarks that are used are without any consent, and the publication of the trademark is without permission or backing by the trademark owner. All trademarks and brands within this book are for clarifying purposes only and are the owned by the owners themselves, not affiliated with this document.

Table of Content

Introduction *1*

Chapter 1: What Is Intermittent Fasting?3

The Science Of Fasting 6

Health Benefits Of Intermittent Fasting 8

Common Myths And Misconceptons About Intermittent Fasting 16

Aging And Intermittent Fasting 21

Chapter 2: Types Of Intermittent Fasting23

Why Should I Try Intermittent Fasting?...... 32

Side Effects Of Intermittent Fasting 34

Tips For Motivation And Success................. 42

More Tips On How To Lose Weight............. 46

Chapter 3: Basic Diet Guidelines...........57

Fluids To Take While Fasting...................... 62

Best Foods You Need To Incoporate Into Your Diet68

Foods To Avoid When Fasting 96

50 Foods With 50 Calories Or Less............. 98

50 Foods With 100 Calories Or Less..........103

Replacement Foods 108

Age-Related Challenges............................. 110

Antiaging 101 113

Savor Your Way To Better Skin 115

Chapter 4: The 21 Day Guide For Fast And Easy Weight Loss 117

The Dawn Phenomenon...........................206

Frequently Asked Questions......................211

A Day In The Life Of Intermittent Fasting . 215

Conclusion.. 217

Introduction

Many things that make weight loss more difficult after age 50 include; decreased appetite, achy joints, diminished muscle mass and even sleep problems. At the same time, losing weight, particularly dangerous belly fat, will significantly reduce your risk of serious health problems such as diabetes, heart attacks and cancer.

Naturally the risk of developing many diseases increases as you age. In some cases, intermittent fasting for women over 50, when it comes to weight loss and reducing the chance of developing usually age-related diseases, may act as a virtual youth pool.

Food fads have come and gone over the last few decades, but the standard medical advice on what constitutes a healthy lifestyle has remained much the same: eating low-fat foods, exercising more... and never, skipping meals. Over that same era, obesity levels have risen worldwide.

So, is there a different approach, based on evidence? One that's based on facts, not opinion? Okay, you guessed it "Intermittent fasting".

When you first heard of Intermittent Fasting's supposed advantages, you were suspicious, as were many. Fasting seems dramatic, daunting-and we both knew that dieting is generally doomed to fail from any explanation. But we're sure of its incredible promise now that we've looked at it in depth and tested it out ourselves. A prominent medical expert once said: 'There is nothing else you can do to your body that is as powerful as fasting.'

Chapter **1**:

What Is Intermittent Fasting?

Fasting in one key sense is completely different to starvation: CONTROL. Starvation is the occasional abstention from eating. It is neither intended, nor regulated. Starving people have no idea when and where they will get their next meal. It happens in times of war and drought, when there is insufficient food. Fasting, on the other hand, is abstaining voluntarily from eating for spiritual, health or other reasons. Food is available freely but you choose not to consume it. No matter what the justification for abstaining, a critical distinction is that fasting is voluntary.

Hunger and fasting should never be confused and the terms should never be used interchangeably. Fasts and hungers live on opposite sides of the world. It's the difference between running and driving, because you're being chased by a lion. External forces impose hunger upon you. On the other hand, fasting can be done for any period, from a few hours to months on end. You can start a fast at any time of your choice, and you can also end a quick at will. For whatever cause, or for no reason at all, you can start or stop a fast.

Fasting doesn't have a traditional duration — because it's just the lack of meals, you're fasting basically whenever you're not feeding. For example, the next day, a span of twelve hours or so, you could fast between dinner and breakfast. Fasting should be seen as a part of everyday life in that way. Take the word breakfast. The word refers to the "break your fast" meal— which is done daily. The word itself clearly recognizes that fasting is done daily, far from being any form of cruel and unusual punishment, even if only for a short duration. It's not a strange thing but a part of daily life.

Although fasting was observed for decades, it was largely forgotten as a dietary therapy. There are basically no books on that. A few websites are dedicated to fasting. Newspapers or magazines make virtually no mention of it. Even its mere name attracts incredulity stars. It is a hiding place in plain sight. Why did they do this?

Big food corporations have been slowly changing how we conceive about fasting through the influence of ads. Rather than being a purifying, balanced tradition, it is now seen as something to be hated and at all costs avoided. Fasting was incredibly bad for business, after all — selling food is hard if people are not going to eat. Fasting has become slowly though ultimately banned. Nutritional officials also say that even missing a single meal will have dire consequences for the wellbeing.

Those advertisements are in books everywhere–on Radio, in the newspaper. Hearing them over and over again creates the illusion that they are certainly absolutely true and scientifically proven. The exact opposite is true. There is absolutely no correlation between healthy eating and good health.

Sometimes the officials will try to convince you, because you will be overcome by starvation, that you can't easy. It's too difficult. It just isn't possible. The irony here is the exact opposite too.

The Science Of Fasting

For most wildlife, festival and drought cycles are the norm. Our distant ancestors often did not eat four to five meals a day. Instead, they will attack, binge, lie about and then have to go without finding anything to eat for long periods of time. In a world of scarcity our bodies and our DNA were forged, punctuated by periodic massive blow-out.

Things are of course very different these days. We're eating something all the time. Fasting—the voluntary abstention from eating food—is seen as something to do that is quite eccentric, not to mention harmful. Most of us expect to eat at least three meals a day, and have snacks between them. They also graze away from the meals and snacks; a milky cappuccino here, the occasional biscuit there, or perhaps a smoothie because it's 'healthier'.

Parents once told their children not to eat amongst meals. Gone are those days. Recent research in the US, which measured the eating habits of 28,000 children and 36,000 adults over the last 30 years, found that the amount of time spent between what the researchers coyly described as 'food times' has dropped by an average of an hour. Or put it another way, the amount of time we spent 'not consuming' has fallen dramatically over the past few decades.

The belief that eating little and often is a 'good thing' has been driven in part by candy makers and faddish diet books, but the medical establishment has also given support. Their argument is that eating lots of small meals is better, because we are less likely to get hungry and gorge on high-fat junk that way. I can understand the point and there have been studies that suggest that eating small meals often has health benefits as long as you don't just end up eating more. But that's just what happens in the real world.

Snacking, in other words, doesn't seem to mean we consume less at mealtime; it just whets the appetite.

Health Benefits Of Intermittent Fasting

1.Intermittent Fasting Changes The Function of Cells, Genes and Hormones

Some things happen in your body when you are not feeding for a while.

For example, the body starts essential processes of cellular repair and adjusts the hormone levels so that accumulated body fat is more available.

- Here are some of the changes that take place in your body during fasting:

- Insulin levels: insulin levels decrease dramatically in the blood, which promotes fat burning.

- Human growth hormone: growth hormone blood levels can increase up to5-fold. Higher levels of this hormone promote loss of fat and gaining muscle, and have many other benefits.

- Cellular repair: The body causes essential mechanisms of cellular repair, such as removing waste material from cells.

•Gene expression: Different genes and molecules have beneficial effects related to survival and disease prevention.

These changes in hormones, gene expression and cell function are linked to many of the effects of intermittent fasting.

2.Intermittent Fasting Can Help You Lose Weight and Belly Fat

Many of those who pursue intermittent fasting do it for weight loss.

The intermittent fasting would usually make you eat fewer meals.

If you make up for it by eating even more during the other meals, you will end up taking less calories.

Therefore, intermittent fasting improves hormone regulation to reduce weight loss.

Lower levels of insulin, higher levels of growth hormone, and elevated concentrations of norepinephrine (noradrenaline) all increase body fat loss and promote the energy usage.

In fact, short-term fasting raises your metabolic rate by 3.6-14 percent, which makes you eat even more calories.

Intermittent fasting, in other words, operates on both sides of the calorie scale. This increases your metabolic rate and reduces the amount of food you eat (reduces calories in).

An intermittent fasting will cause weight loss of 3-8 percent over 3-24 weeks, according to a 2014 analysis of the scientific literature. That is an enormous amount.

Women have lost 4-7 per cent of their waist circumference, meaning they lost lots of belly fat, the unhealthy fat that causes disease in the abdominal cavity.

One research study also showed that intermittent fasting resulted in less muscle loss than a prolonged limit on calories.

3.Intermittent Fasting Can Reduce Insulin Resistance, Lowering Your Risk of Type 2 Diabetes

Over recent decades, type 2 diabetes has become incredibly prevalent.

The main feature in terms of insulin resistance is high blood sugar levels.

Anything that increases exposure to insulin will help reduce blood sugar levels and protect against type 2 diabetes.

Ironically, intermittent fasting has been shown to have significant benefits for insulin resistance, leading to a remarkable reduction in blood sugar.

Fasting blood sugar has been lowered by 3-6% in human studies on intermittent fasting, while fasting insulin has been decreased by 20-31%.

Only one study in diabetic rats found that intermittent fasting helped against kidney damage, one of the most serious diabetes complications.

What this means is that intermittent fasting for people at risk of having type 2-diabetes can be highly protective.

There may be some gender differences, however. One female study showed that blood sugar control actually worsened after an intermittent fasting protocol that lasted for 22 days.

4.Intermittent Fasting Can Reduce Oxidative Stress and Inflammation in The Body

One of the steps towards aging and many chronic diseases is oxidative stress.

This includes unstable molecules, called free radicals, which react to and destroy other essential molecules (such as protein and DNA).

Many studies show that intermittent fasting can improve the body's oxidative stress tolerance.

Furthermore, studies show that intermittent fasting may help combat inflammation, another key driver of common diseases of all kinds

5.Intermittent Fasting May be Beneficial For Heart Health

Heart disease is one of the biggest killers in the world right now.

It is understood that different health indicators (so-called "risk factors") are either associated with an elevated or diminished risk of heart disease.

Numerous different risk factors including blood pressure, HDL and LDL cholesterol, blood triglycerides, inflammatory markers and blood sugar levels have been shown to boost intermittent fasting.

Much of this is therefore based on animal experiments. There is a need to study the effects on heart health much further in humans before recommendations can be made.

6.Intermittent Fasting Induces Various Cellular Repair Processes

The cells in the body start a cycle of cellular "waste removal" called autophagy, when we fast.

It involves breaking down the cells and metabolizing the damaged and defective proteins that over time build up inside the cells.

Improved autophagy can guard against several diseases, including cancer and Alzheimer's disease.

7.Intermittent Fasting May Help Prevent Cancer

Cancer is a terrible disease which is marked by unregulated cell growth.

Fasting has been shown to have some beneficial effects on metabolism which could lead to reduced cancer risk.

Given the need for human studies, encouraging data from animal studies suggests that intermittent fasting may help to prevent cancer.

There is also some evidence for patients with human cancer which suggests that fasting has reduced various side effects of chemotherapy.

8.Intermittent Fasting is Good For Your Brain

What is good for the body is good for the brain too.

Intermittent fasting improves the different metabolic characteristics that are considered to be critical for brain health.

It entails diminished oxidative stress, lowered inflammation, and increased levels of blood sugar and resistance to insulin.

Several rat studies have shown that intermittent fasting will stimulate the growth of new nerve cells, which should improve brain function.

It also raises rates of a brain hormone called neurotropic brain-derived factor (BDNF), a lack of which has been associated in depression and numerous other brain issues.

Animal studies have also shown that intermittent fasting by stroke protects against brain damage.

9.Intermittent Fasting May Help Prevent Alzheimer's Disease

Alzheimer's disease is the most common neurodegenerative disease in the world.

There is no treatment available for Alzheimer's so it is important to keep it from occurring in the first place.

A rat study showed intermittent fasting can delay the onset of Alzheimer's disease or decrease its frequency.

A dietary change that included regular short-term fasts could significantly improve Alzheimer's symptoms in 9 out of 10 cases in a series of case reports.

Animal studies also show that fasting will guard against other neurodegenerative diseases, including disease caused by Parkinson and Huntington.

10. Intermittent Fasting May Extend Your Lifespan, Helping You Live Longer

One of intermittent fasting's most promising uses could be its potential to prolong lifespan.

Studies in rodents have shown that intermittent fasting increases lifespan in a similar fashion to constant restriction of calories.

The results had been quite severe in some of these trials. In one of them, rats that fasted every other day lived 83 per cent longer than non-fasted rats.

Though this is far from being proved in humans, intermittent fasting among the anti-aging crowd has become very common.

Given the known metabolic benefits and all kinds of health markers, it makes sense that intermittent fasting would help you live longer, healthier lives.

Common Myths And Misconceptons About Intermittent Fasting

There are a lot of misconceptions when it comes to intermittent fasting and it is imperative to clarify these myths.

1.Intermittent fasting slows down metabolic rates: Research has shown that daily meals improve metabolism, although this is valid it is also important to note that intermittent fasting does the same as well. Evidence has shown that intermittent fasting improves the metabolism of the body by 3.6-14 percent; although other factors will decide whether you lose weight.

2.Intermittent fasting causes muscle loss: Muscle loss can only result when intermittent fasting is done incorrectly; when done correctly you will not lose your muscle as long as you eat enough protein. You will not weaken muscles or atrophy when you eat a balanced diet and pair it with resistance training because you are consuming the glycogen stored in the body.

3.Fasting lowers your testosterone levels: This is a little more complex as research has shown that extended fasting decreases testosterone levels but, after weeks of fasting, it rises to a higher level. The testosterone levels increase exponentially, with shorter fasting times (24 hours). Evidence has shown that, in fasting, testosterone increases exponentially 20-30 more than in a fed environment. The reason for the testosterone increase is because fasting is a form of stress on the body. Stress stimulates the levels of cortisol that cause testosterone production, as well as the elevation of the growth hormone that keeps the muscle mass.

4. The brain needs a regular supply of dietary glucose to function: There is a misconception that your brain will stop working if you don't eat carbs every few hours, because the brain needs glucose for food. This is completely untrue because glucose is created by the body through a process called gluconeogenesis. The body produces ketone from dietary fats during extended starvation, or very low carbohydrates diets. Ketone acts as a glucose substitute and this makes the brain less glucose dependent.

5. Easting regularly is good for your health: Short-term fasting helps the body rebuild old and damaged cells and is termed autophagy in this process. Autophagy helps protect against tumors, mortality and Alzheimer's disease. Evidence has shown that daily snacking affects your wellbeing and increases your chance of getting sick. Research have shown that high-calorie foods increase your

chances of liver fat and people who eat more have an increased risk of colorectal cancer.

6.Intermittent fasting is bad for your health: You may have learned that intermittent fasting is bad for your health, but tests have shown quite the contrary. It has been proven that it affects the expression of your gene which is responsible for survival and immunity. It is also good for metabolic health, insulin sensitivity, reducing oxidative stress, heart disease and inflammation. This improves brain health by increasing the neurotropic factor (BDNF) produced in the brain, a hormone that protects against depression and other mental health disorders.

7.Intermittent fasting is a form of starvation diet: When you miss a 24-48 hour meal you're not going to starve. Tests have shown you need to run for more than 60 hours straight before the metabolic rate of resting decreases. Starvation is famine-caused suffering or death. The fat reserves in the body become exhausted through malnutrition and the body needs to break down the muscle tissue for nutrition. The fat stored in the body is released during intermittent fasting, and the muscle and lean tissue are untouched. Unless it's an intense extended fast and the fat levels are below 4 percent, intermittent fasting won't affect either muscle or lean tissue as long as it's done correctly with a dietitian or doctor's assistance.

8.When you are not fasting you can eat whatever you like: It's important to note that when you fast, you won't lose weight if you exceed the amount of calories you consume during your off days. It is recommended that you eat a balanced diet which includes fruits, vegetables and whole grains. You can try fish, lean meat, eggs, beans, poultry and nuts without any dietary restrictions.

9.Intermittent fasting is bad for women: This is a frequently asked question by women and expert studies have been contradictory. During intermittent fasting, premenopausal women will experience changes in their hormones but this only occurs when there is a sustained fast. Many women might not tolerate intermittent fasting because they are more prone to depression and it is quite difficult. There are women who run every day for 20 hours, and do not undergo hormonal changes. It depends largely on the woman's genetic makeup, as some can well respond to stress associated with intermittent fasting while others cannot endure it. It is best to start small and increase the intermittent fasting times slowly so the body can gradually adjust to the changes.

10.Gorge and assume you will still lose some fat: Intermittent fasting is very successful on reduction of weight. There's no need for regular checks; all you need to do is stop eating processed foods and stick to regular healthy meals.

Aging And Intermittent Fasting

For years, people have been searching for the key to remain young, healthy and fit. In 2018, the worldwide anti-aging industry contributed US$ 42.51 billion, and by 2023 is projected to reach US$ 55 billion. No one has discovered the elusive cure to fend off depression, weight gain, joint pain, and all the rest not so fun side effects of getting older, despite a lot of money funneling into science and rising consumer spending.

Intermittent fasting has well-documented age-related advantages, in addition to potential positive effects on the brain. There are various ways in which extended fasting helps slow down the aging process. The first is mild inflammation. Research has shown that IF is associated with a decreased inflammation of the brain, and other experiments have seen the effect in other tissues.

Inflammation is a biological defense mechanism, which occurs naturally when the immune system identifies threats such as a compromised enzyme, poisonous agent, or pathogen. However, if inflammation kicks up too often or gets out of control, it can lead to chronic inflammation across the body, resulting in tissue damage or illness. In a 2016 literature review, an analysis of how inflammation is caused and discussed found that too much can cause cardiovascular disease, atherosclerosis, type 2 diabetes, rheumatoid arthritis and some cancers. In brief, keeping inflammation under balance using IF may be able to keep us safe longer.

The second process through which IF tends to delay ageing is by reducing the aggregation of molecules weakened by free radicals, according to the study. Free radicals are radioactive molecules which can kill cells and cause aging and disease.

Chapter 2:

Types Of Intermittent Fasting

The 16/8 Method

This is one of the most common methods that you can use in intermittent fasting. During this method you have to fast for about 14 to 16 hours each day, and eat the rest of the hours. During this feeding time, you can still take in two to three meals with no problem. This is more likely to fit in with the lunch schedule that you're used to, but it still affects you so you don't eat all day.

This approach is simpler than you'd expect. After dinner it's as easy as not eating meals and then skipping breakfast or at least having a late snack. Okay, you're just fasting for 16 hours because you're finishing your last meal at 8 o'clock in the night, and then eating nothing until midday the next day. Just be careful of the late-night therapies. Eating them in the morning will require you to skip coffee.

Many people have issues with this because in the morning they feel hungry for food and they know they need to sleep. Only shift the meal to a bit later in the day. If you choose, for example, to eat breakfast at 10 a.m. You would still be within the 16-hour period instead of eight, and then stop eating at 6 a.m.

As a woman, this form of intermittent fasting is advisable. With these shorter fasts, women typically do well and it is best to go fasting for 14 to 15 hours as this is more helpful to you.

During the quick, you are allowed to drink beer, tea, coffee and other non-caloric liquids to help lessen hunger pains. In fact, you should try to stick to healthier foods during your feeding time. Eating a lot of unsanitary food during this time isn't a good idea. Many people like to have a low-carb diet when they are on a fast intermittent because it deals with fatigue and gives better outcomes.

The rationale behind the approach of 16/8 focuses on your hormonal rhythms and biological clock. According to Satchidananda Panda, a professor at the Salk Institute for Biological Studies and an expert in the field of biology and circadian rhythms, the body has not only one biological clock but several which make up the full circadian rhythm. There's one biological clock in your liver, one in your kidneys and one in your stomach, and according to Panda, each of these clocks were switched on and turned off at various times.

Shortly after you feed the digestive system kicks in gear. When food moves through your digestive tract, every organ involved in the digestive process turns on, eats the food, and then turns off. When all digestive organs are shut off, it will allow the digestive system time to rest. During this time, the digestive system does its own "cleanup"— similar to a concept of a self-cleaning oven. Any remaining food residues are cleaned out, and the body is ready to start over again.

And if you constantly put food in your mouth, it will never shut down your digestive system, so it will never have enough time to perform its self-cleaning, which will have a negative impact on both your metabolism and overall health. Through his study, Panda found that giving the body an eight to twelve-hour, no-food window is best for your health. He claims it will help you lose weight (or maintain a healthy weight) and help stave off diabetes, high cholesterol and obesity by introducing a daily fasting period.

The Importance of Your Circadian Rhythm

For fully understand Panda's work, it is helpful to know what your circadian rhythm is, and how it affects the body. Also referred to as a body clock or biological clock, the circadian rhythm is a twenty-four-hour cycle that regulates many of the body's physiological processes, including sleep and digestion.

The body gets signals from your circadian rhythm about when to go to sleep, when to wake up and when to feed.

Your circadian rhythm is regulated centrally by a brain area called the hypothalamus but is primarily influenced by natural, environmental signals such as temperature and light. For example, when it's dark outside, your eyes send a signal to your hypothalamus that it's time for you to sleep; your hypothalamus sends a message to the pineal gland (in another area of your brain) that activates melatonin (a hormone that helps you sleep), and you get sleepy. When it is light-out the opposite happens. Your eyes send your hypothalamus a signal, sending a signal to your pineal gland to reduce the production of melatonin. A dip in melatonin will make you stand up and get ready for the day.

The 5:2 diet

The 5:2 diet is another viable option. This fast advises you to eat normally for five days during the week and to limit yourself for each of the other two days to no more than 600 calories. This is sometimes called the Easy Diet, too.

It's recommended that on these fasting days, people will eat around 500 calories. You'll normally eat every day of the week, for example, and on Monday and Thursdays you'll have only two small meals with at least 500 calories. You can choose any day of the week as your fasting days, as long as you don't have them back to back. Choose your two busy days of the week, and make them fasting days.

There aren't many reports out there about the 5:2 diet, but it will provide most of the benefits you're finding as it's intermittent fast. You can do it without the need to think all day about making meals.

Eat-Stop-Eat diet

The Eat-Stop-Eat diet helps you skip 24-hour meals once or twice a week. This method was first popularized by Brad Pilon and has been a popular way to do the sporadic quickly for some time. You can do this quickly while still having one meal a day. Some citizens will have dinner every day, and then eat nothing until the supper of the next day. It lets you never go a whole day without eating but still collapsing in the 24-hour abstinence process.

You do want to change that though. You can choose one of those options when going from breakfast to breakfast or lunch to lunch is best for you. During your fast, you are allowed to have coffee, water, and other non-caloric drinks to keep you hydrated but you are not permitted to have any food at all.

Note that you're just fasting for one or two days a week. If it's time to eat properly, you need to consume the same amount of food you would have if you weren't on a fast. This will help you lose weight without hurting your body.

The only problem with getting on with this kind of erratic fast is that working for 24 hours is hard for most people. Nonetheless, you can ease that in it. You can find that beginning with a shorter speed, like the 16-hour fast, can produce some good results, and then continue to run for longer periods of time. Without food it can be hard to go through a whole day and most people tend to go with one of the other fasting options to see the same effects.

Alternate day fasting

With this choice, -alternate day you'll go on a fast. You can take with you a few things, and it depends on what applies to your needs. Some of those fasts that would allow you to have around 500 calories on your fasting days. You will find that most sporadic laboratory studies used some version of the simple alternate day to help determine all health benefits. Every other day it can be daunting to most people to fast.

It's certainly something you'll need to build up to every other day. It can be a struggle to push yourself to eat on alternate days. You'll probably feel very hungry many days a week on this fasting schedule, and it's hard to stick to that over the long run.

Warrior Diet

This is another popular option to choose from for intermittent fasting. This involves eating small amounts of raw fruits and vegetables during the day, followed by a large evening meal. It requires that you walk the entire day, eat just enough to keep you happy and then feast at night within a four-hour feeding window. The Warrior diet is one of the first diets to include a form of intermittent fasting.

Food choices which mimic the Paleo diet are also included in the warrior diet. Not only are you going to fast during most day and night events, but you are going to eat a diet full of unprocessed foods that look like what you see in nature.

Spontaneous Meal Skipping

You should do this if you want to prep your body for intermittent fasting, or if you don't want to spend a lot of time worrying about when you can drink. With this easy, you don't need to worry about following one of the more organized, intermittent fasting programs. You'll probably miss any meals occasionally. If you are not thirsty, or if you are too exhausted for a meal, you can do this. It is a big myth that you have to eat food every few hours to stop hunger.

The liver is well adapted without food, to last long periods. Waiting on a few meals isn't harmful to your health, particularly if you're not hungry or too busy.

If you end up eating a meal, or two, you are actually fasting. If you are too busy to get a snack out of the door just make sure you eat a good lunch and dinner. When you run out of errands and can't find a place to eat, then it's great to miss out on a snack. It will do no good and will really save you money.

You probably won't see results as good as some of the other options, but it's better than nothing and it's much easier to work with. Perhaps try skipping one or two meals during the week, or missing any meals when it's going for you.

As you can see, there are several different options you can deal with when you're ready to go on the sporadic quick. Some of these will be simpler than others and some will fit your timetable better. You'll need to choose which pace to work in your everyday life is best.

Extended Fasting

Although extended fasting belongs to one class of its own, it is important to understand the difference between it and the other types of intermittent fasting. Extended fasting is any form of fast that lasts longer than 24 hours. Long fasting can often last for a week and many of these long fasts simply require drinking liquids.

These types of fasts are more normal throughout the medical and surgical settings and are usually done when the body needs to experience substantial recovery or when the ability to feed is impaired. Without the guidance and monitoring of a medical professional, you should not pursue a continuous pace.

Why Should I Try Intermittent Fasting?

1.Reduces insulin resistance: Fasting is one of the most effective ways to restore the insulin receptors to a normal level.

2.Autophagy: This is the wonderful way the cells can "eat themselves" to get rid of damaged cells and replace the younger elements. Autophagy is also the mechanism by which foreign invaders such as viruses, bacteria, and other organisms are killed. Another method is apoptosis on regeneration of the whole cell. Without this process, the cancer risk increases, as damaged cells continue replicating.

3.Detoxification: Most of us have had prolonged access to diet and climate pollutants. Most of those are contained in our bodies ' fat cells. Fasting is one of the most powerful ways the body can absorb toxins.

4.Circadian Rhythms: The internal clock of your body regulates almost every process in your body and a cascade of negative effects can occur when it is disrupted. You reset the circadian clock, if you take a break from feeding.

5.Gut health: Fasting gives you the opportunity to refresh your digestive system and gut flora. This is significant, because the health of your digestive system regulates your immune system. There's more and more evidence that our moods and mental health co-depend on our gut microbiome.

6.Weight loss: Not necessarily, weight loss is improved by fasting. It also decreases insulin levels so the body won't receive the warning to retain extra calories as fat any more.

7.Brain Function: When you don't eat, your body burns up your blood and liver reserves of glucose and then the liver turns fat into ketones and starts to use them for fuel. In addition, the brain and heart prefer ketones to fuel glucose, because they create less harmful reactive oxygen species (ROS). Your brain should work better and improve your reasoning and learning ability.

8.Heart function: With their high energy demands the heart cells can use fats, sugars, ketones and amino acids. Ketones have a metabolic role in fine tuning that optimizes cardiac output and protects the heart from inflammation and injury.

Side Effects Of Intermittent Fasting

- If you're always worried about what to eat next, it could be a sign of orthorexia.

Dieting can generally lead to orthorexia, a disorder involving an obsession with eating healthy. Some of the signs of orthorexia include the need to talk all the time about your diet, and a concern for your next meal.

- Intermittent fasting can disrupt your sleep, which is critical to health.

There is some preliminary evidence that by preventing you from waking up in the middle of the night, intermittent fasting will enhance sleep. Their feeding time often appears to close just before they go to bed as people start their fast sooner. It makes them avoid snacking during the night which can improve sleep quality.

- If you lose your period or experience hair loss, it could be related to fasting.

Intermittent fasting can cause a calorie deficit in some individuals, which can result in hair loss and erratic or missing hours. With low blood sugar, people on an intermittent fasting diet may also feel colder than normal.

- Feeling hangry

We're not 100% positive "hangriness" is a real word, but it's definitely a real feeling. That's the sensation of grouchiness, grumpiness, or general irritability that comes with being unable to sleep while your body tells you it's thirsty.

When previously reported by WH, preparing the body to go 16 hours without food takes some practice, and within a limited timeframe, the bodies of some people may not ever be comfortable feeding.

By principle, you shouldn't be hungry first thing in the morning if you eat enough protein later in the day or night. But if you are, that's a warning that during your caloric intake cycle you need to make some nutritional changes to avoid turning into a big crank — or it's an indication that fasting just doesn't vibrate well. Never eating for long periods may not be suitable for some people (e.g. those who work out a ton)—and that's definitely something worth remembering.

There are some drinks or spices allowed on fasts that can help suppress hunger.

- Water: Start the day with a full glass of cold water. Staying hydrated aids in avoiding hunger. (Before dinner, drinking a glass of water can also minimize nausea and help prevent overeating.) Sparkling mineral water can assist relieve loud stomachs and cramps.

•Green tea: Full with antioxidants and polyphenols, green tea is a great dietary aid. The potent antioxidants can help boost metabolism and weight loss.

•Cinnamon: Stomach emptying has been shown to be sluggish and may help alleviate hunger. It can also help to lower blood sugar and is therefore helpful in losing weight. For a delightful change of pace, cinnamon can be added to all the teas and coffees.

•Coffee: While many believe that caffeine in coffee suppresses appetite, tests have shown that this effect is more likely to be linked with antioxidants— although caffeine that increase the metabolism, fat burning may also improve. However, a study shows that both decaffeinated and regular coffee suppresses the hunger in water better than caffeine. There is no reason to limit coffee intake due to its health benefits.

•Chia seeds: rich in soluble fibers and omega-3 fatty acids. Such beans, when immersed in liquid for thirty minutes, absorb water and form a gel which can assist in suppressing appetite. They can be consumed dry or made into a pudding or gel. These may be taken to help alleviate hunger during a fast. Also, although breaking the fast technologically, the effect is so small that it does not distract substantially from the advantages of the quick. The improved enforcement more than makes up for it.

•Fatigue or brain fog

Have you ever found yourself yawning over and over the middle of the morning, only to realize that you have never had a breakfast before? Since not eating breakfast is typically the way most people do IF, realizing that you're excessively tired every day— or making stupid mistakes because you're wading through brain fog — is a tip-off that you don't eat the right food during non-fasting hours, or that fasting doesn't fit your lifestyle requirements.

•Low blood sugar

During IF, if you're experiencing constant nausea, headaches, or dizziness, that's a red flag suggesting the diet can throw your blood sugar out of whack. As previously reported by World Health Organization, diabetics should for this very reason stop some form of fasting diet: IF can cause you to become hypoglycemic, a risky state for anyone with insulin or thyroid problems.

•Hair loss

While intermittent fasting doesn't necessarily lead to a nutrient loss, eating a well-rounded diet tends to be harder when you cram a whole day worth eating in a few hours. When you find that every day more hair falls out in the bathroom than normal, re-evaluate the nutritional content of your daily meals and talk to your doctor about whether intermittent fasting is a wise move for you.

•Changes in your menstrual cycle

Here's another side effect of sudden weight loss (which can be due to IF): women who lose a dramatic amount of weight or who consistently don't get enough calories every day may find their menstrual cycles slowing down or even stopping altogether.

People who have unusually low body weight are vulnerable to a condition known as amenorrhea, or menstrual absence. Sudden weight loss or underweight may interfere with your typical hormone cycle and cause missed periods; so while you may be happy about how IF has helped you shed pounds, you may also deprive your body of the calories it needs to work.

Start fasting and speaking to your gynecologist for troubleshooting if you stop getting your period and suspect it's due to intermittent fasting practices you're practicing.

•Constipation

It's easy for people to fail to drink water during hours of fasting, she says, but going 16 hours a day without enough liquids is a (gastrointestinal) catastrophe formula. So if you've begun an IF diet and you don't seem to be able to get your bowel movements to happen regularly (or at all), it's time to pause on your program to talk to a nutritionist or MD about what's going on (in this situation, or not!).

•Unhealthy diet

Even though IF does not cause a serious disorder such as orthorexia, it could still lead to some pretty unhealthy eating habits. Besides not getting the proper nutrients, during non-fasting hours you might also find yourself making messy nutritious choices.

•Feeling Cold

Cold fingers and toes are quite common while fasting but for a good reason! If you fast, the supply of blood to your fat stores decreases. Called blood flow of adipose tissue, this helps move fat into your muscles, where it can be burnt as a fuel. You can also make you more susceptible to feeling cold while your blood sugar is through. Beat coldness by sipping hot tea, enjoying warm showers, adding extra layers and avoiding extended periods of time outside in the cold.

•Bathroom Trips

If you drink enough oceans to stay hydrated and fill you up, you can feel the need to run more often to the toilet. We think about it perhaps even twice an hour! I'm sorry to say around this there's no way. You certainly don't want the water consumption to be limited, so make sure you're still close to a toilet.

Breaking Your Fast

Break your fast gently. The longer the time of fasting, the gentler that you have to be. There is a natural tendency to overeat as soon as the fast is over— although, surprisingly, most people say this is not because of sheer appetite but rather because of a subconscious need to eat. Eating too much right after fasting often leads to discomfort in the stomach. It can be quite unpleasant though not extreme. The problem appears to be self-correcting.

Try to start breaking your fast with a snack or a little dish, then wait thirty-sixty minutes before eating your main meal. Normally this will give you time to push through any waves of hunger and allow you to slowly begin to eat again. Short-lasting fasts (twenty-four hours or less) usually do not require special preparation but it is a good idea to plan ahead for longer fasts. Prepare a small dish and leave it in the fridge to be ready and less likely to be tempted by the myriad of other convenience foods available when it comes to breaking the fast.

Tips for Breaking Your Fast with a Snack

- •Make sure that the size of your portion is small. You're going to eat a full meal soon so there's no need for gorge.

- •Take time to do extensive chewing. This will improve the digestive system, which has been sleeping for a while, tremendously. You bring your system back online slowly.

- •As a general rule, take your time. Your speed is finished. If you feel anxious to eat again, be comfortable knowing that in the hour you will have a whole lunch.

- •Don't forget water to drink! Before breaking your fast and after your first meal, drink a tall glass of water! People often forget to eat food after they avoid fasting but we often confuse hunger thirst. Make sure that you stay hydrated so that you do not over-eat.

Tips For Motivation And Success

Try to avoid the temptation to sabotage: One of the things that can make your efforts at intermittent fasting to be futile is if you give in to the temptation of foods in your fridge or pantry. If you easily succumb to food on first sight, then it is advisable to shop every few days for groceries rather than stocking up weekly or bi-weekly. If you happen to stay with your family, you can ask them to hide any tempting foods away from you.

1. Organize your fridge to make your fasting days easier: Arrange your fasting day foods to one section of the fridge as this helps you to train your eyes and mind to search for only foods that you want to eat on your fasting days. With time your eyes and mind won't wander all over the fridge looking at foods you aren't allowed to eat.

2. Socializing doesn't have to involve food: Food is one of the things that unite family and friends, and it is embedded in our culture. Regardless of this, there are other fun things that you can do on your fasting days that doesn't involve food when you are out there socializing. By concentrating on those activities, you can take your mind off food but be careful so that you don't become a hermit while fasting.

3.If you are a trigger eater, try and overcome such triggers: Everyone has something that triggers us to eat. For examples; during break time at work you may be triggered to go to the vending machine while watching TV you may want to have a drink or some snack, or maybe you pick leftovers while clearing the dishes; regardless of what the trigger is you have to find a way to overcome such triggers. Before you begin with your intermittent fasting, make sure to note all the times you snack and find a way to deal with those triggers. During your break time at work, you can decide to go for a ten-minute walk, have another person clear the dinner table, do some needlework, cut coupons, do some stretching or chew a piece of gum while watching TV.

4.Set up a reward system: The best way to complete a major goal is to set smaller goals and celebrate them when you have achieved it. When you complete a set of fasting days, or you lose a pound, you can give yourself a little treat. You can buy yourself a new book, get a manicure, watch a movie with a loved one at the cinema or hang out by yourself at the park.

5.Get your family and friends to join you on your intermittent fasting plan: Let your family and friends know about the intermittent fasting plan you want to embark on and give them the guidelines. Even if they don't partake in the program, they can give you words of encouragement and motivation by telling you how great you look or not showing up at your house with foods that you have stopped eating.

6.Find a partner: If can find a partner to intermittent fast with you, it can serve as a good source of motivation. Find a family or friend that would love to try the 5:2 fast diet so that you can mutually support and encourage each other.

7.Don't rush: Learn to take it one day at a time: Don't overthink about how you will survive the month as this can overwhelm you. You can try to think of it like this, "I don't have to stick to my diet tomorrow; I just have to get through today." Say this to yourself every day, and you will get through it.

8.Understand your body: If you can tell the difference between hunger and other feelings, you will avoid mindless eating. Most of our mindless eating happens because we are angry, bored, or tired. Try and study your feelings any time you feel like grabbing a snack. To take your mind off it, you can either try to talk to your friend on the phone or go to bed.

9.If you feel the urge to eat try and drink some water: It might be tough to tell the difference between thirst and hunger, but anytime you feel the urge to get a snack, try and drink a glass of water. You may be surprised that the urge to eat may disappear more often than not.

More Tips On How To Lose Weight

1.Learn to enjoy strength training

While cardio gets a lot of attention when it comes to weight loss, strength training is also important for older adults in particular.

Your muscle mass declines as you age, in a process called sarcopenia. This muscle mass loss starts around the age of 50 and can slow down your metabolism which can lead to weight gain.

Your muscle mass declines by around 1–2 percent per year after age 50, while your muscle strength decreases at a rate of 1.5–5 percent per annum.

To reduce age-related muscle loss and promote a healthy body weight, adding muscle-building exercises to your routine is therefore necessary.

Strength training, such as workouts on body weight and weightlifting, will greatly improve muscle strength and increase muscle size and function.

Furthermore, strength training can help you lose weight by reducing body fat and boosting your metabolism, which can increase the amount of calories you are burning all day.

2.Team up

It can be difficult to put in a healthy eating habit or workout schedule on your own. Pairing with a friend, coworker or family member may give you a better chance to stick to your plan and achieve your goals for wellness.

Research, for example, suggests that those completing weight loss programs with peers are considerably more likely to sustain their weight loss over time.

Working with friends can also reinforce your commitment to a fitness program and make the exercise more enjoyable.

3.Sit less and move more

Burning more calories is important to removing excess body fat. That's why it is important to be healthier all day while trying to lose weight.

Sitting at your job for long periods of time, for example, can hinder your attempts to lose weight. To combat that, simply by getting up from your office and taking a five-minute walk every hour you can become more involved in the job.

Research shows that monitoring the steps using a pedometer or Fitbit will improve weight loss by raising the activity levels and calorie expenditure.

Start with a practical progress target based on your current activity levels when using a Pedometer or Fitbit. Then work your way steadily up to 7,000–10,000 steps per day or more, based on your overall health.

4.Bump up your protein intake

It is not only necessary to get enough high-quality protein in your diet for weight loss but also essential to avoid or reverse age-related muscle loss.

How many calories you consume at rest, or your resting metabolic rate (RMR), declines per decade after turning 20 by 1–2 percent. This is associated with muscle loss associated with aging.

Eating a diet high in proteins, however, will help prevent or even reverse muscle loss. However, numerous studies have shown that growing dietary protein can help you lose weight and hold it off over the long run.

However, research shows that older adults have higher protein requirements than younger adults, which makes adding protein-rich foods to your meals and snacks all the more important.

5.Talk to a dietitian

It can be difficult to find an eating pattern that both encourages weight loss and feeds on your body.

Consulting a registered dietitian will help you figure out how best to remove excess body fat without having to follow an overly restrictive diet. Furthermore, a dietitian will help and guide you on your path to weight loss.

Research shows that partnering with a dietitian to lose weight can lead to considerably better results than doing it alone, and it can help you keep the weight loss going through time.

6.Cook more at home

Several studies have shown that people who prepare and consume more home-made meals tend to follow a healthier diet and weigh less than those who don't.

Cooking meals at home allows you to monitor what's going into your dishes— and what's left out. It also helps you to play with good, special ingredients that pique your interest.

When you eat most meals out of the house, begin by cooking one or two meals a week at home, then raise this amount slowly until you cook more than you eat out at home.

7.Eat more produce

Vegetables and fruits are packed with nutrients which are vital to your health, and adding them to your diet is a simple, evidence-based way of reducing excess weight.

For instance, a study of 10 studies found that every daily vegetable serving rise was correlated with a 0.14-inch (0.36-cm) reduction in women's waist circumference.

Another survey of 26,340 men and women aged 35–65 contributed to eating lower body weight fruits and vegetables, decreased waist circumference and less body fat.

8.Hire a personal trainer

For fact, training with a personal trainer will help someone new to working out by showing you the best way to exercise and encourage weight loss and avoid injury.

Besides, you may be motivated by personal trainers to work out more by keeping you accountable. We can even improve your fitness behavior.

A 10-week research of 129 adults found that one-on - one personal training for 1 hour per week improved fitness motivation and raised levels of physical activity.

9.Rely less on convenience foods

Eating convenience foods daily, such as fast foods, sweets, and fried snacks, is correlated with weight gain and may impede the weight loss efforts.

Convenience foods tend to be high in calories and poor in important nutrients such as fat, sugar, vitamins and minerals. That is why fast foods and other processed foods are generally referred to as "empty calories." Reducing convenience foods and substituting them with nutritious meals and snacks based around nutrient-dense whole foods is a good way to lose weight.

10. Find an activity you love

It can be difficult to find an exercise routine that you can maintain over the long term. That is why engaging in the activities that you enjoy is important.

For starters, if you like group activities; sign up for a local sport such as soccer or a running club so you can do regular exercise with others.

If solo workouts are more of your type, try your own run, stroll, climb or swim.

11. Get checked by a healthcare provider

If you are struggling to lose weight even if you are involved and follow a healthy diet, it may be advisable to rule out factors that may make it difficult to lose weight — such as hypothyroidism and ovarian polycystic syndrome (PCOS).

This can be especially true if you have members of your family with those conditions.

Inform your healthcare provider about your problems so that they can agree on the right testing protocol to rule out medical conditions that may be behind your weight loss challenges.

12. Eat whole-food-based-diet

One of the simplest ways to make sure your body gets the nutrients it needs to thrive is by following a diet rich in whole food.

Whole foods, including vegetables, bananas, nuts, beans, meat, fish, legumes, and grains, are filled with essential nutrients to maintain a healthy body weight, such as calcium, protein, and healthy fats.

In many trials, the weight loss has been linked with whole-food diets, both plant-based diets and those that contain animal products.

13. Eating less at night

Several studies have shown that eating fewer calories at night can help you keep your body weight healthy and lose excess body fat.

A study with 1,245 people found that those who consumed more calories at dinner over 6 years were more than 2 times more likely to become obese than those who ate more calories earlier in the day.

Additionally, those who ate more calories at dinner were considerably more likely to develop metabolic syndrome, a group of conditions including high blood sugar and excess belly fat. Metabolic syndrome increases your risk of developing heart disease, diabetes and stroke.

Eating most of the calories through breakfast and lunch, while eating a lighter meal, may be a successful weight loss process.

14. Focus on body composition

Although body weight is a good indicator of health, your body composition is also important— meaning the percentages of fat and fat-free mass in your body.

Muscle mass is a significant indicator of overall health, especially for older adults. Your goal should be to add on more muscle and shed excess fat.

There are many ways to measure a proportion of your body fat. Actually weighing your hips, biceps, ankles, chest and thighs will help you determine if you lose fat and gain muscle.

15. Hydrate the healthy way

Drinks such as sweetened coffee beverages, soda, juices, sports drinks and premade smoothies are often packed with calories and added sugars.

Drinking sugar-sweetened beverages is strongly linked to weight gain and conditions such as obesity, heart disease, diabetes and fatty liver disease, especially those sweetened with high-fructose corn syrup.

Swapping sugar beverages with healthy drinks such as water and herbal tea can help you lose weight, and can significantly reduce your risk of developing the above mentioned chronic conditions.

16. Pick the right supplements

When you feel tired and unmotivated, taking the right supplements will help you get the strength you need to achieve your goals.

As you get older, your ability to absorb those nutrients reduces and the chance of malnutrition becomes increasing. Evidence, for example, indicates that adults over 50 are generally deficient in folate and vitamin B12, two nutrients required to produce electricity.

Deficiencies in B vitamins such as B12 will adversely affect your mood, induce fatigue and hinder weight loss.

For this cause, consuming a high quality B-complex vitamin to further lower the risk of deficiency is a good idea for those over 50 years of age.

17. Reduce added sugars

Limiting high added sugar products, including sweetened beverages, chocolate, desserts, biscuits, ice cream, sweetened yogurts, and sucrose cereals, is vital to weight loss at any age.

Since sugar is applied to so many foods, including things you wouldn't suspect like tomato sauce, salad dressing, and pizza, reading ingredient labels is the best way to determine whether an item has added sugar.

Search for "added sugars" on the label with nutrition facts, or check for popular sweeteners like cane sugar, high-fructose corn syrup, and agave ingredients chart.

18. Improve the quality of your sleep

Not getting enough quality sleep can damage your efforts to lose weight. Several studies have shown that inability to get enough sleep increases the likelihood of obesity, and may discourage attempts to lose weight.

2-year survey of 245 women, for example, found that those who slept 7 hours per night or more were 33% more likely to lose weight than those who slept less than 7 hours per night.

Better quality of sleep was also correlated with success on weight loss.

Try to get the required 7–9 hours of sleep per night and improve the quality of your sleep by reducing the light in your bedroom and stop using your phone or watching television until bed

19. Be more mindful

Eating mindful can be a simple way to improve your food relationship, all while encouraging weight loss.

Mindful eating means paying more attention to your dietary habits and food. It gives you a better understanding of your signs of hunger and fullness, and how food affects your mood and wellbeing.

There have been many studies that using careful eating techniques promotes weight loss and improves eating behaviors.

There are no specific rules for eating conscientiously, but feeding gently, paying attention to the scent and taste of each bite of food and keeping track of how you feel during your meals are simple ways to incorporate healthy eating into your life.

Chapter 3:

Basic Diet Guidelines

You don't get as many calories to eat when you reach 50, as you do in your 20s. This ensures you have even less space to make unhealthy choices. Calorie needs vary depending on age, but a sedentary 50-year-old woman needs about 1,600 calories a day just to maintain her weight, while a slightly more active woman requires 1,800 and an active woman will need about 2,000 to 2,200 per day. Meet your calorie needs by eating more whole, less-processed foods such as fruit, beans, whole grains, lean protein options and low-fat dairy foods to keep your weight in check and fend off disease.

Energize With a Good Breakfast

Whole grains are a great way of energizing your day. According to the Academy of Nutrition and Dietetics, whole-grain fiber may help lower your risk of colon and prostate cancer. A healthy breakfast option could include a bowl of unsweetened whole grain cereal topped with fresh fruit such as a banana or non-fat milk blueberries, or a full wheat English muffin breakfast sandwich, scrambled eggs made with two egg whites and one egg yolk and a slice of low-fat cheese. Serve the sandwich with cantaloupe slices and a cup of nonfat milk.

Load Up on Fruits and Vegetables at Lunch

Fruit and vegetables are low in calories and filled with nutrients that contribute to disease control. You need at least 4½ servings of fruits and vegetables a day but you can strive for nine. Another way to help you fulfill your everyday vegetable needs is to add a lean protein like turkey or fish, dried fruit and low-fat salad dressing. You can also add a stir-fry to your vegetable intake, like shrimp sautéed with broccoli, celery and carrots and served with brown rice and an orange.

Meat as a Side Dish at Dinner

The Academy of Nutrition and Dietetics says eating too much meat raises the risk of heart disease and colon cancer. Make meat a side dish to help you cut back, and consider the vegetable and whole grains the main attraction. A nutritious dinner may include, for example, a big baked potato with grilled asparagus and a side of grilled beef tenderloin. And, to make you eat more seafood, prepare tacos of tuna filled with grilled peppers, onions and salmon and be eaten on the cob with corn.

Foods for Hormone Support

You can sound as though the emotions are on a roller-coaster ride in midlife. Hot flashes, night sweats and mood swings are just a few of the peri-menopause and menopause side effects that usually occur at age 50. Eating more healthy fats will help you manage the effects should you feel them. Omega-3 fatty acids exist in cold water fish such as salmon, sardines, and tuna. Flaxseed is a good source of alpha linolenic acid, a kind of omega-3, dependent on plants. These tiny seeds also provide lignans, a variety of fibers that can reduce hot flashes. The omega-3s help heart health as an extra bonus, another concern for women aged 50 and over.

Soy products such as soy milk, tofu, miso, edamame and tempeh contain isoflavones, which are natural compounds that imitate the body's hormones and can help ease the symptoms of menopause. However, if you're a breast cancer survivor, eating lots of soy may not be acceptable— if that's you, talk to your doctor before you add it to your diet.

Foods for Bone Health

In the middle age women's bones became thin, leaving them vulnerable to fractures and osteoporosis. To help bone health the body depends on calcium and vitamin D. Among the best calcium food sources are dairy products such as cow and goat's milk, cereal, and cheese. Calcium is also produced by broccoli, collards and turnip greens, almonds and Brazil nuts, soy crops, and blackstrap molasses. Vitamin D is better obtained by small amounts of exposure to the sun, but it is also supplemented with fish, cod, egg yolks, soy milk and some fortified cereals and juices. You may also take supplements formulated with vitamin D.

Foods with Antioxidants for Aging

Foods containing antioxidants help prevent free radicals, which are rogue molecules formed during the natural aging process and by exposure to toxins from the environment. Free radicals disrupt the normal cells and DNA as you age, diminishing the ability to fend off diseases like cancer.

Increasing your consumption of high in antioxidant fresh fruits and vegetables will improve your defenses. Vitamin C is a strong antioxidant that comes with citrus fruits, lettuce, bell peppers, parsley, salmon, kiwi and tomatoes. Another is vitamin E present in peas, almonds, whole grains and vegetable oils which are cold-pressed. Beta-carotene, or provitamin A, is obtained from a wide variety of purple, red, and orange vegetables such as cabbage, onions, sweet potatoes, cantaloupe, and peaches, and green vegetables such as broccoli, kale, and spinach. The mineral selenium, present in brewer's yeast, wheat germ, Brazil nuts and whole grains in particular, acts with vitamin E to fulfill antioxidant roles in the body.

Fluids To Take While Fasting

While fasting, only certain fluids can be consumed like; water, tea, and coffee (hot or iced) and homemade broth.

•WATER: The benefits of water cannot be overemphasized, so you must drink water frequently throughout the day when you fast. You can enjoy flat, mineral or carbonated water. You can add;

>•You can add lime

>•You can add lemon

>•You can add slices of other fruits (never eat the fruit or consume fruit juice)

>•You can add vinegar (raw, unfiltered apple cider vinegar is better)

>•You can add Himalayan salt

>•You can add Chia and ground flaxseed (mix one tablespoon in a cup of water

•You can add sweetened powders or drops

•COFFEE: Consuming up to six cups of their caffeinated or decaffeinated coffee is allowed. Black coffee is preferable, but you are only allowed to add one tablespoon of certain fats to each cup of coffee taken. You can also have a change by taking unsweetened iced coffee. Brew your coffee and then refrigerate it or add ice cubes.

•You can add coconut oil

•You can add medium-chain triglyceride oil (MCT oil)

•You can add butter

•You can add Ghee

•You can add heavy whipping cream (35% fat)

•You can add half and half milk

•You can add whole milk

•You can add ground cinnamon, for flavor

•Try and avoid low fat or skimmed milk; whole milk is preferable

•You can add powdered dairy products

•You can add natural or artificial sweeteners of your choice

•HERBAL TEA: There is no limit as to the number of herbal tea you can consume during your fasting period. There are quite a number of herbal teas that can help suppress your appetite and lower your blood sugar levels.

•Green tea: This serves as an excellent appetite suppressant

•Cinnamon Chai tea: This helps to lower the blood sugar levels, and it is also useful for suppressing cravings of sweet food.

•Peppermint tea: This acts as an excellent appetite suppressant. It helps with alleviating GI discomfort, such as gas and bloating.

•Bitter melon tea: It helps to lower blood sugar levels

- Oolong tea: This also helps to reduce blood sugar levels

Black tea is preferable, but you are only allowed to add one tablespoon of certain fats to each cup of coffee taken. You can also have a change by taking unsweetened iced coffee. Brew your coffee and then refrigerate it or add ice cubes.

- You can add coconut oil

- You can add medium-chain triglyceride oil (MCT oil)

- You can add butter

- You can add Ghee

- You can add heavy whipping cream (35% fat)

- You can add half and half milk

- You can add whole milk

- You can add ground cinnamon, for flavor

- Try and avoid low fat or skimmed milk; whole milk is preferable

- •You can add powdered dairy products

- •You can add natural or artificial sweeteners of your choice

•HOMEMADE BROTH: It is normal if you experience some lightheadedness during the first few days of fasting. This is caused by dehydration and low levels of electrolytes, and it can reduce by taking a good homemade broth. Both vegetable and broth made with meat, fish, or bones will work. Bone broth is very beneficial because it contains an essential ingredient called gelatin which is very good for people who have arthritis or other joint problems. There is no limit as to the amount of broth you can consume during the fasting day.

- •You can mix any vegetable that goes above the ground

- •You can take leafy vegetables

- •Carrots

- •Onions or shallots

- •Bitter melon

•Animal meat

•Animal bones

•Fish meat

•Fish bones

•Himalayan salt

•Any dried or fresh herbs and spices

•One tablespoon of ground flaxseed per cup

•Vegetable puree of any kind

•Potatoes, yam, beets or turnips

•Always avoid any store-bought broths even though they
  are organic

Best Foods You Need To Incoporate Into Your Diet

1.Oats

The risk of heart disease increases dramatically in women over 50, so it's a smart move to add more cholesterol-lowering items such as oats into your diet. Oats are abundant in a form of soluble fiber called beta glucan and it has been shown that eating at least 3 grams of this fiber per day (equivalent to 1.5 cups of cooked oatmeal) lowers HDL and LDL cholesterol levels by 5 to 10 per cent. People who regularly eat oats and other whole grains often face a reduced risk of early death. For other healthy ingredients such as almonds, beans, and fruit, plain oats are cheaper than canned cereals and a natural conduit.

2.Apples

We are definitely not as beautiful as acai berries or mangosteen, but apples are as excellent as exotic fruits, and much, much cheaper. A big apple contains 5 grams of heart-healthy fiber, and research shows that regular eating apples will reduce both HDL and LDL cholesterol and help keep the ticker in tip-top shape. A study conducted in 2013 showed that chronic apple eaters posed a lower risk for type 2 diabetes. And the good news is, apples can be found nearly everywhere, including gas stations and convenience stores. Slice one up and add a peanut butter smear to a classic snack that will never get stale.

3.Nuts

Snacking on almonds instead of popcorn, crackers and biscuits is a simple way to deliver a major upgrade to your diet. A 2013 randomized controlled trial in Spain found that eating an ounce of mixed nuts daily as part of a Mediterranean diet decreased the risk of heart attack, stroke, and heart disease mortality by 28%. And don't forget that peanuts do count — they're just as good, but they cost only half as much as almonds and other tree nuts. Another easy way to get into a routine service: using brown rice and quinoa as a garnish with roasted vegetables or whole grain sides.

4.Leafy Greens

Piling on the lettuce, broccoli, collards, or other leafy greens at meals will help keep your mind healthy as you mature. According to studies discussed last month at the American Society for Nutrition annual meeting, people who ate one or two meals per day had the same cognitive ability as people 11 years younger who never eat the greens. Cooking greens needn't be difficult. Take a baby spinach bag for a hassle-free side dish and sauté the leaves whole in an olive oil drizzle with optional chopped garlic. Heads up: If you are taking coumadin thinner in the blood, you don't have to give up completely on greens; talk to your doctor about adjusting your medication to allow for small portions of it every day.

5.Berries

Protect against: Cancer, diabetes, heart disease, memory loss, and obesity

Key nutrients: Anthocyanins, antioxidants, fiber, and vitamin C

It's incredible what eating only a handful of berries can do for your health. Those who eat 1 cup of blueberries a week had a 23 per cent reduced risk of developing diabetes in a study involving 200,000 men and women. With ½ cup of blueberries or 1 cup of strawberries a week, elderly women's brains (with an average age of 50) were protected from age-related memory decline. Researchers at Harvard claimed the berry eaters postponed their cognitive decline by as much as 2½ years.

Anthocyanins tend to be the "magic" ingredients in the berries responsible for these benefits — red and blue pigments that are strong antioxidants. Such compounds were also related to a reduced risk of a number of cancers. On top of that, each type of berry comes with its own nutritious bonus: Blueberries have the lowest anthocyanin concentration. Raspberries have the most fiber — at 8 grams per cup, more than any other fruit ounce for ounce. One cup of strawberries has more vitamin C in a day than one requires. Cranberries have five times broccoli's antioxidant strength, and they're a natural probiotic, which means they'll raise good bacteria rates and shield you from foodborne diseases. Blackberries can help to reduce cholesterol and blood pressures and can play an important role in the prevention of diabetes, heart disease and cancer. And berries are the least calorie-rich in all fruits, between 53 and 84 strawberries per cup.

While berries are delicate and their season is short, fresh berries can be frozen for up to one year or packed frozen ones can be purchased. Also look out the names as some brands come loaded with sugar. Cranberries are so tart in their natural state that cranberry goods are often dreadfully oversweetened. You will buy fresh cranberries even cooler for making your soup or smoothie.

6.Yogurt

Eating adequate protein distributed throughout the day will help maintain the muscle and slow down the gradual decrease in lean body mass that happens as our bodies' age. Yogurt, particularly Greek varieties, at breakfast and snack time can provide a generous dose of high-quality protein, the times of the day when we tend to eat carbier meals. Cow's milk yogurt and fortified non-dairy varieties are also good sources of calcium, a vitamin required by women over the age of 50 to preserve bone health in greater quantities. And the beneficial bacteria that lend its tang to yogurt may also help to nourish the stomach. Purchase the simple stuff and substitute it with nutritious mix-ins such as fresh or dried fruit, almonds, vegetables, whole grain cereals, or (for a treat) dark chocolate chips to keep added sugar to a low.

7.Beans

Protect against: Diabetes, heart disease, and obesity

Key nutrients: Antioxidants, folate, potassium, protein, and soluble fiber

We all know the old adage about beans, but they're literally good for your heart— and also for the rest of your body. We are food world chameleons, capable of performing a number of culinary functions. Beans will act as a protein, a "healthy" carb and even a serving of vegetables.

Soluble fiber is one of their most important products. Beans have more of the compound than virtually any other substance. Soluble fiber absorbs water in your digestive tract, so it gradually exits your stomach and has a beneficial effect on your weight (because you stay more full longer) and blood sugar levels. In a National Health and Nutrition Review survey study, scientists found that people who eat beans were 23 per cent less likely than those who never ate beans to have wide waists. And researchers at the University of Toronto found that people with type 2 diabetes who ate mostly low-glycemic-index foods such as nuts and beans improved their blood sugar levels and were at lower risk of heart disease than those who ate mostly whole grain breads, cereals, and brown rice.

Soluble fiber often interferes with dietary cholesterol absorption, so it can reduce the cholesterol levels in your body. Scientists at Mesa's Arizona State University Polytechnic found that adding ½ cup of beans to soup decreases cholesterol levels by as much as 8 percent.

Black beans, red kidney beans, and other dark-colored beans in antioxidants are as high or higher as vivid fruits and vegetables. But this doesn't mean paler beans don't have any appeal. White beans, for example, give you 100 milligrams of calcium per ½ cup-a decent number! So lentils are one of the best sources of B vitamin folate, which is so significant in decreasing birth defect risk and also plays a role in the health of the heart and brain.

Sadly, the rest of that childhood chant— the line that rhymes with heart— is real, too. Beans contain complex, non-digestible sugars called oligosaccharides. We are fermented in your stomach by the good bacteria, which cause gas and bloating. Yet both of you can reduce oligosaccharides in beans to make your body more immune to them. Beans soaking overnight and then boiling them in fresh water or rinsing canned beans will help remove the sugars. (Rinsing canned beans often eliminates around 40 percent of their salt, so it's a good idea whether you're suffering from bean-related bloat or not.) Drink plenty of water while you eat beans (or any other high-fiber food), and begin with small portions so that your digestive system changes. This way, without the unpleasant consequences, you get the health benefits.

8.Apples

Protect against: Heart disease, high cholesterol, obesity, and stroke

Key nutrients: Antioxidants and soluble fiber

It's time to step up your apple IQ! Not only are apples among the most versatile, inexpensive, and genuinely diverse fruits (with 7,500 different types, there's an apple for every taste preferences, from sweet to tart), they're both true health powerhouses. The strength of their fiber makes apples extremely rewarding. In one study, at a meal, people who crunched 15 minutes before a meal ate 15 per cent fewer calories. This turned into a shortfall of 60 calories, until you add in the apple calories. That may not sound like much, but if you did it once a day you would almost effortlessly lose 6 pounds over the course of a year.

Approximately one-third of apple fiber is soluble which is the form that helps to lower cholesterol. To achieve this effect you need 3 to 5 grams of soluble fiber a day; a medium apple has 2 grams. And apples also keep your cardiovascular system ticking along in another way: they are rich in antioxidant flavonoid quercetin and anti-inflammatory polyphenol compounds. A Dutch study found that having one medium apple a day could reduce your risk of stroke by about 43 per cent.

9.Asparagus

Protects against: Bloating, cancer, digestive upset, and obesity

Key nutrients: Folate, glutathione, inulin, and saponins

Try switching out the celery sticks for asparagus spears the next time you're eating vegetables and dip. The beautiful crop is hard to beat when it comes to nutrient density. Seven large spears provide 72 percent of your daily vitamin K— a nutrient required for blood coagulation and bone health — for a measly 28 calories. You also get 3 grams of fiber in the form of cancer-fighting carotenoids, 20 percent of your daily vitamin A, 18 percent of your folate, 17 percent of your calcium, and some vitamin B6 and vitamin E.

Asparagus is a good source of three difficult-to-find compounds in many foods: inulin, glutathione, and saponins. Inulin is a fiber type that possesses prebiotic properties. That means it serves as fuel for the healthy bacteria in your intestinal system, a feature likely to be responsible for the reputation of asparagus as a folk remedy for digestive woes.

Asparagus is known to be a leading anti-inflammatory food due in part to its high glutathione content, which some scientists find to be the most potent antioxidant. This compound improves the infection-fighting capabilities of your immune system, and also helps to repair cell damage, which is often a first step in cancer growth. Saponins are phytochemicals which can help lower the cholesterol and reduce the risk of cancer.

While there are no studies to prove this, it is said that asparagus has a diuretic effect, and may help ease bloating. Combined with its high-fiber and low-calorie count, these properties mean that asparagus is a good diet to consume while you try to lose weight. Many people claim asparagus often alleviates hangovers. One small study found that asparagus extract improved the ability of the liver to process alcohol and protected the liver cells from the damage that alcohol can cause — but that was in the test tubes. So go ahead and stick your Bloody Mary in an asparagus knife, if you like. When you indulge in one too many, just don't allow it to shield you from a banging heart.

10. Avocados

Protect against: Cancer, diabetes, heart disease, macular degeneration, and obesity

Key nutrients: Beta-carotene, fiber, folate, lutein, monounsaturated fat, phytosterols, potassium, and zeaxanthin

Ever notice that you scarcely have space for your tacos when you have guacamole as an appetizer? That's because avocados are packed with a potent combination of fiber and healthy fats— there are 8 grams and 18 grams in ½ cup of guac, respectively! Including the fluffy green fruit (yes, avocados are a fruit) will keep you feeling satisfied with your dinner. A research at California's Loma Linda University showed that people who had half an avocado created more leptin— the fullness hormone— for up to three hours after they fed.

Two-thirds of the avocado fat is monounsaturated, helping to lower insulin levels and to facilitate weight loss. What's more, a mono-rich diet actually lets you shed belly fat.

Monounsaturated fats provide a number of other health benefits: they reduce inflammation, cholesterol, triglycerides, and blood sugar, and prevent deteriorating memory related to age. Monos also help to keep skin plump and smooth by replenishing the protective layer of fatty acids that retain fluids that cover skin cells.

Avocados are also the best source of phytosterols in the crop, compounds that alter the way the body processes cholesterol and can help lower rates of LDL (or "bad"). And avocados are filled with B vitamin folate, essential for heart health and birth defect prevention, as well as carotenoids such as beta-carotene, lutein, and zeaxanthin. These antioxidants add to healthier eyes and guard against cancer and heart disease. What's more, avocados help you consume more of these antioxidants at the same time from any other foods you eat. Researchers served lettuce, cabbage, and spinach salads on men and women in a report from Ohio State University. The participants consumed 8.3 times the alpha-carotene when the salad contained avocado, 13.6 times the beta-carotene and 4.3 times the lutein they did when they ate an avocado-free salad.

There has to be a trap with so many perks, right? Okay yeah, but it's a slight one: Avocados ' high fat content also means they are high in calories relative to other fruits and vegetables. A middle-sized avocado has 114 calories in just one half. So look out for the portion sizes and have your guac instead of chips of crudites.

11. Broccoli

Protects against: Cancer and heart disease

Key nutrients: Fiber, folate, sulforaphane, and vitamin C

Criticized by a president and millions of picky eaters, broccoli has a reputation for being an unpleasantly smelling bitter-tasting vegetable. But that's not the fault of broccoli-blame the chef! Too often broccoli is overcooked, leaving it an appetizing, drab color, rendering it mushy, and trapping the compounds of sulfur that are responsible for some of its strong flavor. If you were a broccoli-hater you owe it to your wellbeing to try again. Broccoli is a real all-star diet along with other members of the cruciferous family, such as cabbage, cauliflower, Brussels sprouts, broccoli rabe, bok choy and turnips.

Let's start with the fundamentals: A cup of broccoli will give you a heavy dose of calcium, manganese, potassium, phosphorus, magnesium, sugar, starch, folate and vitamins C and K. It has 3 grams of protein, as well. The cancer-fighting compounds of broccoli include carotenoids, and particularly sulforaphane. Japanese scientists found that women with breast cancer who ate lots of broccoli and other cruciferous vegetables cut their risk of recurrence by 35 percent and their chances of dying from the disease by 62 percent over a 3-year period. The saddest thing about overcooking broccoli is it kills a lot of the nutrients. To reap the advantages of broccoli and learn to love it, blanch it for a few minutes in boiling water, or steam it until it turns bright green. That is when you know this food is soft enough but still crunchy enough to love. Serving broccoli with whole grains or nuts will help soften the bitterness, as well as mixing it with sweeter vegetables such as red peppers, carrots or caramelized onions. Stir-frying garlic broccoli does that trick too. Consider broccolini if all else fails, which has a comparable nutritional profile but a milder, peppery flavor.

12. Dark leafy greens

Protect against: Cancer, diabetes, macular degeneration, and obesity

Key nutrients: Calcium, carotenoids, fiber, folate, iron, vitamin C, and vitamin K

Nutritionists like to talk about "nutrient density": the amount of nutrients that you get from a meal compared to its calorie count. Among the most nutritious foods on the world are the mild-tasting roman lettuce and spinach, the peppery arugula and mesclun, the slightly acidic escarole, cabbage, Swiss chard, and collars, calories for calories, dark leafy greens. For example, 1 cup of cooked kale contains 1.327% of your daily vitamin K, 354% of your daily vitamin A (in the form of antioxidant carotenoids), 89% of your vitamin C, 9% of your calcium, 8% of your iron and potassium, 6% of your magnesium, 4% of your folate and vitamin E, and 3 grams of fiber. It also includes sulforaphane— a drug that battles cancer present in cruciferous vegetables. All this just for 36 calories. All the leafy greens (even iceberg lettuce) produce the same nutrients to one degree or another. But the greener the darker the more nutritious it is. Iceberg fans, try romaine: It has the same soothing texture, but carotenoids 9 times, vitamin C 7.5 times, folate 4 times, and vitamin K 3.6 times.

A carotenoid content makes dark leafy greens effective cancer fighters as well as defensive against pain. Lutein has been linked to a lower risk of macular degeneration (the leading cause of blindness) and cataracts, a carotenoid abundant in greens. Vitamin K is an effective anti-inflammatory medication and some studies suggest it helps prevent inflammation from developing. It is a major component of bone health, too.

Some of the deepest-hued greens ' strong flavors make people shy away from them but you can do a few things to make them more palatable. Blanch strong greens such as kale and collars in boiling water until the hue is vivid, around 2-3 minutes. Then sauté the vegetables in a savory olive oil with garlic. In salads, the milder-tasting vegetables can be mixed with peppery ones.

Apprendre to love greens is worth the effort. According to a report from the Harvard Nurses ' Health Study, having only one serving a day (1 cup of raw greens or ½ cup of cooked) cuts your heart attack risk by around 23 percent. More is better: Italian researchers found that women eating 2 ounces of greens a day (about 1½ cups of raw spinach or 1 cup of chopped raw kale) lowered their chances of developing heart disease by about 46 per cent. And a Leicester University study found a strong correlation between dark leafy greens and a reduced risk of type 2 diabetes. Those who ate at least 1½ servings a day were 14% less likely to develop the disease, something that the researchers attribute to the high levels of greens magnesium. Need some extra incentive? Scientists at Munich University found that people scored around 20 percent higher on a novelty test when they got a preview of the green color beforehand. We claim that our brains equate the color with nature, which allows us to think about development and growth. So throw yourself a dark green salad the next time you feel uninspired.

13. Mangoes

Protect against: Diabetes, digestive problems, heart disease, and obesity

Key nutrients: Carotenoids, fiber, vitamin C, and vitamin E

The next time someone complains that "healthy food is bland and boring," give the person a mango what happens. Nice, juicy, tropical mangoes taste luscious and decadent but are among the healthiest fruits in the world. For one study, people who ate 1¼ cups of mango daily for a month reported a 37 percent drop for levels of triglycerides, which helps to reduce risk of heart disease. Another heart-healthy mango perk is that it contains the antioxidant vitamin E. The antioxidant carotenoids in mangoes not only make them a good source of vitamin A, supplying 36% of your daily needs in just 1 cup, but they also help protect against cancer.

Mangoes make a tasty side dish with chicken, pork, or fish topping and produce enzymes that help your body break down the protein in these foods. Only one cup contains 10 per cent of your fiber needs. Both of these substances promote digestion.

While the work is preliminary, mangoes can increase fat burning. Scientists at Oklahoma State University in Stillwater found that mice who had been fed mangoes for 2 months as part of their diets weighed the same as mice who had not, but had less body fat and higher blood glucose levels. The body produces less insulin while glucose is small-a drug that can improve fat storage. Low glucose means lower diabetes risk, too.

14. Nuts and nut butters

Protect against: Alzheimer's disease, heart disease, and obesity

Key nutrients: Calcium, healthy fats, magnesium, protein, and vitamin E

The list just keeps growing when it comes to the nutritional benefits of the nuts. They even raise your brainpower while strengthening your spirit. A study published in the journal Neurology found that older people who ate diets high in vitamin E and omega-3 fatty acids were less likely to have cortical shrinkage and more likely to do well on verbal exams than those who did not. And those almonds that you used to eat? From their calorie count you should deduct about 30 percent, as USDA scientists have found that they only have 129 calories an ounce, not 170. The study carried out by the same group also found pistachios to be lower in calories. The pattern is likely to apply to all nuts.

Yet nuts were considered to be big players in weight control even before this work was published, due to the healthy fats, protein, and fiber they all provide in one little box. In a test at Harvard University, participants who had breakfast walnuts remained full all morning and ate fewer calories at lunch time. So nuts will rev your metabolism. Researchers at Georgia Southern University in Statesboro have found that having a high-protein, high-fat snack increases calorie burning more than 3 hours later!

Also, when eating nuts it is possible to go overboard. Measure a part of 1-ounce-about ¼ cup of nuts. Try buying unshelled nuts and opening them yourself, if one batch leads to another. According to a study published in Appetite, noshing on pistachios that you have to shell yourself can help to reduce by more than 40 percent the number of calories you take in. This is presumably because cracking the nuts makes you more mindful of how much you eat and slows you down, allowing your brain room to be pleased with your appetite.

Each nut has its own unique nutritional advantage. Almonds are a decent source of calcium, walnuts are filled with cardio-protective omega-3s and just one Brazil nut more than fulfills the normal selenium need, a mineral that can help protect against cancer. Both nuts contain antioxidants, but they do have the most pecans. As is true with fruits and vegetables, consuming a variety of nuts is better than eating only one kind. You might try to keep a tub of mixed nuts for a quick snack at your desk or in your pantry. Just be sure to keep an eye on your serving size, because nuts are not low in calories.

15. Olive oil

Protects against: Bone loss, cancer, heart disease, obesity, and stroke

Key nutrients: Antioxidants, monounsaturated fat, and vitamin K

Mediterranean cuisine's cornerstone, olive oil is at least partly responsible for the health benefits of the diet— but only if you pick the right type. Any olive oil is a great source of monounsaturated fat but it takes a little thought to get one with many other beneficial compounds. Do not focus on labels to choose the healthiest oil but trust the taste buds. True cold-pressed extra virgin olive oil has a slightly bitter, peppery flavor (the kind to buy for both flavor and health). You will experience a little stinging in the back of your throat or the need to cough as you drink it straight; this is an indication that the oil is high in anti-inflammatory agents, polyphenols and antioxidants.

Olive oil, when as fresh as possible, is at its most therapeutic and flavourful. Heat, breeze, and time reduce the beneficial compounds in the oil, so avoid the labels packaged in clear bottles, never buy an olive oil that doesn't have a "best before" stamp and a date a few months away, and don't be fooled at the warehouse store by the sale on the 5 gallon tank. You should only buy as much as you'll use in a couple of months. Natural olive oil is not inexpensive but it is no guarantee of quality that a high price is. Try to buy your olive oil at a shop that will let you try it in advance (or give it back if you don't like it), and note that a little goes a long way.

Now that you know how to pick the good stuff, this is why olive oil should be a favorite for both frying and drizzling in your oven. That will make your heart full, for one thing. Monounsaturated fats prevent LDL ("bad") cholesterol from oxidizing, a process that leads to clogged arteries. For one study, people who drank the most olive oil had a 44 percent lower risk of dying from heart disease (and a 26 percent lower risk of dying from any cause) than those who eat the least olive oil during the study period. French researchers found that cooking and eating extra virgin olive oil reduces the risk of strokes by 41 per cent. While a group of Spanish scientists researched the impact of Mediterranean diet on heart disease, they found that elderly men who consumed olive oil had a drastic increase in blood markers indicating bone structure, while those who adopted a Mediterranean-style diet of nuts and no oil or low-fat diet did not.

Another reason to store on olive oil: the polyphenols and antioxidants found therein have antibacterial properties which destroy the ulcer-causing bacteria. It has also been shown that certain compounds guard against various cancers.

Finally, foods high in monounsaturated fat help you burn fat in your belly and olive oil is no exception. It seems more rewarding than other fats, too. Scientists at State College's Pennsylvania State University find that a meal cooked in olive oil leaves you healthier than the very same food cooked in corn oil. In Urbana-Champaign, food specialists at the University of Illinois gave 341 Italian restaurant patrons equal quantities of bread and either olive oil or butter. On every slice of bread, the olive oil party ate 26 per cent more fat, but the butter eaters ate more bread and absorbed only 17 per cent more calories.

The message here, however, is not to put olive oil on everything. Calories in olive oil are quickly added up to 120 per tablespoon, so be sure to measure.

16. Quinoa

Protects against: Cancer, diabetes, heart disease, and obesity

Key nutrients: Antioxidants, fiber, folate, iron, magnesium, phosphorus, and protein

Despite gluten-free diets gaining popularity at your local supermarket, you may have noticed a new addition to the grain aisle: quinoa (pronounced KEEN-wah). Yet quinoa isn't really fresh at all; it was once a staple food for Inca warriors, who coveted the grain for their energy-giving properties.

Quinoa isn't really a plant, though it cooks like one, definitely. It is a seed that is botanically similar to beets and Swiss chard, and has some special nutritional properties among "grains." For one thing, it is higher in protein, and that protein is full, ensuring it has all eight essential amino acids, just like eggs and meat do. Both grains contain antioxidants, but quinoa is especially filled with quercetin and kaempferol, anti-inflammatory compounds that are associated with lower cancer risk and heart disease. Quercetine is a popular antihistamine, as well. Quinoa helps balance blood sugar like whole grains, because it has a low glycemic index and is high in fiber. It makes it worthwhile for weight control and treatment of diabetes.

There are also culinary benefits. Quinoa is more nutritious and tasty than brown rice and it cooks in only 15 to 20 minutes. Like smooth, chewy foods, quinoa is both delicate and crunchy. The seed germ twists out and forms a crunchy "tail" when you cook it. It tastes good hot or cold, can be used in sweet or flavorful dishes, and comes in three colors: ivory, red, and black. Take some processing of rice or pasta, and add it in quinoa.

17. Tea

Protects against: Arthritis, bone loss, cancer, diabetes, heart disease, obesity, stroke, and viral infections

Key nutrients: Caffeine and catechins

Tea definitely delivers a potent health punch for a tea that has such a calm, meditative, and somewhat fussy image. The different tea varieties — white, green, oolong, and black— all produce antioxidant polyphenols that are considered catechins. EGCG, present at the highest concentration in green tea, is the most strong of those. Studies have linked regular green tea intake with lower risk of colon, breast, gastric, lung and prostate cancer. A research at London's Kingston University tested 21 plant and herbal extracts, and found white tea to be the most effective in reducing inflammation, decreasing the risk of rheumatoid arthritis, certain tumors, and wrinkles.

EGCG is an aid of metabolism, too. USDA researchers found that people were eating an additional 67 calories a day when they were drinking oolong tea instead of the same amount of caffeinated coffee. We conclude that something in the tea other than caffeine, the catechins most definitely, stimulates the body to burn fat first for energy (rather than carbohydrates). When research participants were drinking tea, fat oxidation was 12 per cent higher. In a small Japanese test, when they drank green tea beforehand, people consumed 17 per cent more fat during a 30-minute exercise.

But black tea every day is not a health slouch, either. According to a study published in the Journal of the American College of Nutrition, people who drink a cup of it after eating high-carb foods drop their blood sugar levels by 10 percent over 2½ hours. Black tea often reduces blood pressure and helps fight LDL ("bad") cholesterol, lowering it in just 3 weeks by up to 10 per cent.

Your immune system is also having a helping hand from tea. Scientists at Pace University in New York City find drinking a cup zaps viruses, such as the ones that cause colds and flu, within 10 minutes. Have you been infected with the sinus? Researchers at the University of Alexandria in Egypt found that green tea enhances antibiotic action, in some cases by threefold. Even sufferers with allergies can get a break: EGCG can block the allergenic response that some people need to pollen, pet dander and dust.

And if all that isn't enough, here's the kicker: Tea will help slow down the bone loss with age. An Australian study found that women between the ages of 70 and 85 who drank tea had greater bone density than women of the same age who did not drink tea.

Herbal tea has not the same antioxidants as standard tea but it has its own health benefits. Chamomile and peppermint, for example, will soothe upset stomachs, passionflower helps you sleep, rosemary wards off stress-induced headaches, and thyme relieves coughing and pressure on the sinus.

When you prepare it yourself, Iced tea is just as strong as hot tea; packaged material varies widely in antioxidant quality. Yet scientists seem unable to agree on the impact that milk has on the antioxidants in tea. Several experiments have shown that milk protein binds the beneficial compounds, but others have shown that it doesn't matter. Drink at least a handful of your cups straight up until the jury exits.

18. Yogurt

Protects against: Digestive problems, heart disease, high blood pressure, obesity, and osteoporosis

Key nutrients: Calcium, potassium, probiotics, protein, and vitamin B12

You probably think of yogurt as a perfect calcium source and you would not be mistaken. (There's only one other product that's a better natural source of this mineral than yogurt, and that's ricotta cheese.) A 6-unce nonfat plain yogurt tub has about 300 milligrams, or 30% of what you need every day.

Yet yogurt is offering so much more. First there's the fat, a big 8 grams, which exceeds the amount in a large egg or ½ cup kidney beans. Greek nonfat yogurt has more protein (18 grams) than regular yogurt but also less calcium (200 mg).

Next is potassium—468 milligrams in 6 ounces, near the quantity in a large banana. Calcium and potassium help to relieve blood pressure. Another study found that two low-fat dairy meals a day reduced 54 per cent of the risk of developing hypertension.

Transforming milk into yogurt involves adding healthy bacteria. For this reason, two strains-Lactobacillus bulgaricus and Streptococcus thermophilus-are used. Many contain L, as well. Acidophilus, a probiotic organism that lives in your digestive tract allows you to stay healthy in a number of ways. (Many yogurt producers add additional probiotic strains to their products.) Probiotics have been demonstrated to boost the immune system. For one study, elderly people who ate about 3 ounces of yogurt a day were 2.6 times less likely than those who did not eat yogurt to catch the colds. Antibiotics lower the number of healthy bacteria in your intestines, which can contribute to diarrhea. Yogurt eating helps you repopulate the good bacteria and reduces your chances of experiencing this unpleasant side effect by around 60 percent. Probiotics are also being researched for their role in preventing and regulating heart disease.

The combination of calcium and protein in yogurt has been shown to make it easier to lose pounds. A research by the Harvard School of Public Health that looked for two decades at the dietary habits of more than 120,000 people found that the intake of nuts and dairy was most closely correlated with the weight loss. Yet yogurt tends to be particularly effective at burning fat in the abdomen. Researchers at the University of Tennessee, Knoxville, found that women who lost weight drinking yogurt had around their waists 81 per cent less fat than those who did not eat yogurt.

All these advantages in terms of weight loss come from drinking plain yogurt. In many ways the sugar-filled material is chocolate for disguise. Some of the sugar in fruit yogurt comes from lactose in the milk itself (anything that ends up with-ose is sugar) or from the fruit itself. Even a plain, unsweetened, low-fat yogurt in a 6-ounce container has 12 grams of sugar. There is no issue with these natural sugars, but fruit and flavored yogurts frequently contain added sugar in the form of sucrose or high-fructose corn syrup. Different brands add different numbers, and both normal and artificial sugars on food labels are lumped together. Buying plain yogurt and adding your own fruit, or even a little honey, if you like, is your best defense. That way, you are regulating how much sugar you consume. Your second best option is to carefully read labels, and pick a flavored yogurt with as close as possible to 12 grams of sugar. If you don't mind substitutes for sugar, yogurts made with them will have the same sugar content as an equal portion of plain yogurt.

19. Dark chocolate

Protects against: Depression, diabetes, heart disease, and obesity

Key nutrients: Flavonoids

You can also have your chocolate, and eat it! Scientific findings have revealed in recent years that this culpable pleasure is in fact a bona fide food for health. Cocoa and dark chocolate, which contain at least 70 percent cacao, are rich in antioxidant flavonoids and are among the highest concentrations of antioxidants in any product. Such antioxidants can provide a variety of advantages including resilience of your arteries and enhancement of your circulation. According to a UK study, people who eat chocolate may be 37 per cent less likely to develop heart disease and 29 per cent less likely to get a stroke than those who don't. And there's evidence that even if you already have heart disease chocolate can be cardio-protective. A Swedish study published in the Journal of Internal Medicines showed that heart attack patients who snacked only twice a week on chocolate were 70 per cent less likely to die from heart problems. The brain profits from more robust arteries too. After drinking a cup of hot cocoa, people in one study were able to count backward faster and more accurately than when they didn't drink cocoa, and they were less likely to feel tired or drained mentally.

Chocolate eaters are also healthier, calmer individuals and, according to a study in the Journal of Proteome Science, regular therapy impacts decrease levels of stress hormones. Certain studies show that the chocolate containing phenethylamine activates endorphin development and contributes to a sensation of well-being comparable to falling in love. For one test, couples were linked, given candy, to brain and heart monitors and then told to kiss. Both the chocolate and the kissing alone made heart pound and brain buzz, but the inclusion of chocolate during the kiss increased excitation levels in the pleasure center of the brain, especially in women.

Paradoxically, giving in to the cravings of candy will make you lose the pounds. For one test, people who had been given pizza 2½ hours after eating dark chocolate ate 15 percent less calories than when they had candy in the milk. Yet researchers at California University, San Diego, conducted a study that made them conclude that chocolate calories are metabolized in such a manner that they do not result in weight gain. Dark chocolate lovers were thinner than those who ate very little of the treat, although overall they did not consume less calories or exert more. You still want the chocolate to stay healthy, so stick to small servings and mix them with other antioxidant-rich foods, such as fruit or nuts.

Foods To Avoid When Fasting

- Potato chips and snack mixes

- Cookies, cakes, and other sweets

- Refined sugar and flours

- Frozen dinners and prepared entrées

- Sugary cereals

- Whole milk and heavy cream

- Flavored yogurt

- Cream-and cheese-based sauces

- Fatty cuts of meat

- Butter or fat for cooking

- Creamy salad dressings

•Sour cream and dip for chips

50 Foods With 50 Calories Or Less

- •1 small apple

- •½ cup of applesauce

- •2 apricots

- •¼ sliced avocado

- •½ cup of baby carrots, with 1 teaspoon light ranch dressing

- •½ small banana

- •1 cup raw of bean sprouts

- •¾ cup of blackberries

- •1 cup of blueberries

- •¼ cup of cantaloupe

- 1 stalk of celery, with ½ tablespoon of peanut butter

- 12 fresh cherries

- 1 Chocolate sandwich cookie

- 8 corn chips

- 1 dark chocolate square

- ½ cup of fresh fruit salad

- 1 all natural of fruit ice,

- ½ grapefruit

- 15 grapes,

- ½ cup of Greek yogurt, 1 teaspoon with of jam

- ½ cup of honeydew, 2 tablespoons with of cottage cheese

- 1 cup of sugar-free hot chocolate,

- 2 tablespoons of Hummus, 2 with carrot sticks

- 20 sugar-free Jelly beans

- 3 cups air-popped of Kettle corn

- ¼ cup of Kiwi

- 1 snack cup of Mandarin oranges

- ½ mango

- 2 large marshmallows

- 1 cup of Miso soup

- 1 cup of raw mushrooms

- 1 small orange

- ½ cup of fresh squeezed orange juice

- 2 slices of oven-roasted deli turkey

•1 Peach

•5 Potato chips

•1 Pretzel rod

•1 cup of radishes, with 1 tablespoon of light ranch dressing

•1 snack box of raisins

•¾ cup of raspberries

•1 plain rice cake

•1 ounce of smoked salmon, with 2 whole-wheat crackers

•8 Strawberries

•1 Tomato, with 1 tablespoon Parmesan

•2 Triscuit crackers

•2 Tuna sushi rolls

- •½ ounce of Turkey jerky

- •¾ cup of Vanilla almond milk

- •1 cup of watermelon

- •3 Whole-wheat crackers

50 Foods With 100 Calories Or Less

- 15 Almonds

- 1 apple, with 2 teaspoons of peanut butter

- 1 cup of unsweetened applesauce

- ¼ sliced avocado, with 1 rice cake

- 2 cups of baby spinach, sautéed with 1 teaspoon of olive oil

- 1 baked apple with cinnamon

- ½ baked potato, with 1 tablespoon of salsa

- 1 small baked sweet potato

- 1 small banana

- 10 Blue corn chips

•3 large carrots

•3 tablespoons of dried cherries

•3 Clementines

•½ cup of cottage cheese, with 1 slice of cantaloupe

•½ cup of cottage cheese, with 4 strawberries

•1 Cucumber, with 2 tablespoons of cream cheese

•3 Dark chocolate squares

•1 slice of Deli turkey, with 1 slice of Swiss cheese

•1/3 cup of Edamame,

•½ of English muffin, with 1 tablespoon of sugar-free fruit
    jelly

•1 small scoop low-fat of frozen yogurt

•¼ cup of all-natural granola

- 1 cup of grapefruit juice

- 30 Grapes

- ½ cup plain of Greek yogurt, with ¼ cup of pureed pumpkin

- 1 Green pepper, with 2 tablespoons of goat cheese

- 1 hard-boiled egg

- 2 tablespoons of Hummus, with 1 cup of baby carrots

- 3 tablespoons of Hummus, with ½ red bell pepper

- 1 Kiwi, with 1 tablespoon of unsweetened shredded coconut

- ¼ cup of Lite Cool Whip, with 12 strawberries

- 1 cup of mango

- ½ cup of mashed potato, with 1 tablespoon of skim milk

- 6 cups of microwave popcorn

- 1 tablespoon of all natural peanut butter

- 1 cup of pineapple

- 30 Pistachios

- 1 mini 100-calorie bag of popcorn

- 40 Pretzel sticks

- 1/3 cup of cooked Quinoa with ground cinnamon

- 2 cups of raspberries

- 3 tablespoons unsalted of roasted soybeans

- 2½ ounces of baked Salmon

- ¾ ounce of sharp cheddar cheese

- 2 medium tangerines

- 2 cups of low-sodium tomato juice

•1 cup of low-sodium tomato soup

•9 mini Tootsie Rolls

•1 cup of low-fat vegetable soup

•2 cups of watermelon

Replacement Foods

•Fresh fruits and vegetables

•Air-popped popcorn with low butter

•Rice cakes and vegetable chips

•Natural sweeteners in moderation. These include honey, maple syrup and more

•Whole grains like quinoa, oats, brown rice, millet, etc.

•Oatmeal or muesli

•Skim milk or non-dairy milk like almond milk, coconut milk, etc.

•Plain nonfat Greek yogurt with fruit

•Vegetable-based sauces

•Lean protein sources like chicken, turkey, fish, shrimp, etc.

•Cooking with vegetable broth

•Vinegar-based salad dressings

Age-Related Challenges

Age-Related Challenges that Hinder Proper Nutrition:

•Decreased sensitivity

As you get older, the senses become numb; it takes more energy and time to activate a sensation. Your sense of smell and taste is increasing your appetite.

You may even have difficulty in some situations separating fresh food from old, because the senses are impaired. That would be unquestionably detrimental to your health.

•Medication side effects

Many medications cause nausea, reduce appetite and alter expectations of the food tastes. The side effects in this situation will prevent you from eating, and you'll end up skipping meals.

•Poor Dental Health issues

Bad dental health problems are more likely to arise as you grow older, such as missing teeth, gums receding that cause weak teeth, mouth sores, and jaw pain.

All of these factors make chewing unpleasant and inconvenient, thereby reducing the likelihood that seniors will take healthy foods.

•Lack of finances

Older people have limited resources and are more worried about money. Therefore, they can cut back on groceries and buy cheaper food which is less nutritious in most cases. This lifestyle will lead to multiple metabolic impairments.

•Lack of transportation

To shop for fresh cooking ingredients, you have to drive to the store, wait for heavy traffic and park your car a short distance from the entrance.

It is even more difficult when it's raining or snowing. Chances of dropping and sliding are high. These may prevent you from shopping altogether.

•Physical challenges

Older people get poorer with age, especially when coping with conditions such as arthritis and disability. Pain and poor physical strength can prove challenging to simple tasks.

Performing basic functions such as long standing when cooking, transporting foodstuffs, or even peeling a fruit can become overwhelming activities.

•Memory loss

Memory loss Memory loss, depression and Alzheimer's disease are quite typical of seniors. A senior may forget to follow their recommended meal program or skip a meal or maybe even forget to buy food from the store. That poses a challenge to diet.

•Depression

As you get older, a lot of changes take place (your kids move on, you miss your friends and loved ones because of death, you feel lonely— especially if you live all alone, you experience physical changes).

Compounding all of these issues can lead to depression. Older people can become apathetic about their health and avoid eating. Depression will lead to far more significant health problems if left untreated.

Antiaging 101

Why is your skin starting to shorten, wrinkle and darken over time? Free radicals from metabolic processes in our bodies or from outside causes such as heat, lack of sleep, fried food, tobacco, air pollution, sun exposure (UV rays), x-rays, smoking cigarettes and chemicals, destroy our skin cells and tissues and cause oxidation. Oxidation happens as free radicals break down elements of a cell, such as their enzymes, DNA, and membranes. Once oxidation happens, the cells lose their proper functioning capabilities. Consider about how a sliced apple is beginning to turn gray. Free radical damage causes youthful thickness of wrinkles in the skin, folds, fatigue, sagging and degradation. Free radicals can cause inflammation, which is not limited to the damaged areas but can also extend to healthy tissue, damaging collagen and elastin, leading to further premature aging, fine lines and wrinkles.

This might sound tragic and futile, but please! Antioxidants can counteract the effects of free radicals, and slow the aging process. Your body can generate certain antioxidants, but its ability to make them reduces as you age. Therefore, packing your diet with anti-aging powerhouse antioxidants such as vitamins A, C and E is important to protect your skin from harm. Furthermore, these beauty boosters increase the development of collagen, restore elasticity, decrease UV damage, reduce inflammation, decrease breakouts and enhance skin texture.

Savor Your Way To Better Skin

Everything you eat and drink contributes to your look and the best news is that it has never been easier or more delicious to eat your way to a youthful glow! Start by feeding your body with anti-aging superstars such as berries, cucumber, watermelon, and tomatoes and you'll quickly look and feel healthier, happier, and more vibrant — from the inside out.

We are always told to drink more water, but are you really aware of why? The cells, muscles, and tissues of our body need to be hydrated to function. Water has a tremendous number of roles: it controls temperature, removes waste, lubricates joints, and carries nutrient relaxation. The equilibrium between the electrolytes and water also determines how well other organ systems work. And, contrary to your beliefs, water isn't just necessary for hydration.

Dehydration, which can simply be caused by a tough, sweaty workout, can lead to a host of problems including dizziness, fainting, fever, heart palpitations, decreased urination, increased heart rate, decreased blood pressure and swollen tongue. (Note: When you notice these symptoms, cool off any way you can, and start increasing your water intake slowly.) Another unpleasant symptom of insufficient water intake is swollen, wrinkled skin. When we mature, the muscles of our bodies cannot retain water just as much as they did when we were younger, and our skin loses the ability to heal itself. But you're going to hydrate your body by drinking at least eight 12-ounce glasses of water a day and reduce the incidence of dried, wrinkled skin.

Try to keep a reusable water bottle on hand (try glass or stainless steel to avoid the harmful chemicals in plastic bottles) if you find it hard to remember guzzling water all day. You should add a few slices of lemon, lime, or cucumber to give a good pop to your water too. There are even flavor-infusing bottles of water which allow you to add fruit and other ingredients to your hydration for a twist.

Chapter 4:

The 21 Day Guide For Fast And Easy Weight Loss

Day 1

BREAKFAST

•Strawberry Banana Pancakes

This pancake is a fun way to give your breakfast a little bit of flavor. Not only is it tasty, it is quick and easy to make too.

Ingredients

•Avocado oil cooking spray

•3 egg whites, lightly beaten

•1 tablespoon almond butter

•1 ripe medium banana, sliced

•4 fresh strawberries, hulled and sliced

•½ teaspoon ground cinnamon

Preparation

•Heat a small frying pan, coated with avocado oil spray over medium-low heat for 1 minute.

•Mix well the egg whites and almond butter together in a medium bowl, and then add the banana and strawberries.

•Pour the mixture into a saucepan, cover the lid and cook for 3 minutes.

•Turn the pancake over the other side for 2 minutes to tan.

•Serve hot, cinnamon sprinkled on top and garnish.

DINNER

•Tangy Orange Chicken Breast

This recipe provides both energy and sweetness. It is a great recipe to whip up at busy nights. It is a light but satisfying meal, served with a green salad and some quinoa or brown rice.

Ingredients

•1 teaspoon of olive oil

•4 (4-to 5-ounce) skinless chicken breasts

•1 teaspoon of paprika

•½ teaspoon of salt

•¼ teaspoon of freshly ground black pepper

•1 teaspoon of fresh thyme chopped

•1 teaspoon of fresh rosemary chopped

•1 teaspoon of unsweetened orange juice concentrate

•2 teaspoons of fresh chopped parsley

Preparation

•Preheat the oven to 400 ° F, and line the aluminum foil baking platter. Apply the olive oil through the pot.

•In a cup, put the chicken breasts, turn over to oil and season with the paprika, salt, pepper, thyme and rosemary.

•Cook for 15 minutes, then turn the chicken and spray the concentrate with the orange juice. Bake for another 15 to 20 minutes, or until the chicken juices are visible.

•Before serving, garnish with parsley;

Day 2

BREAKFAST

•Salmon Omelet

This savory omelet is full of fatty acids called omega-3. It's sure to become a staple of breakfast.

Ingredients

•2 tablespoons olive oil

•¼ cup trimmed and chopped scallions

•1 cup trimmed and chopped asparagus

•1 tablespoon chopped fresh dill

•6 ounces canned salmon

•6 large eggs, beaten

Preparation

- •Mix the olive oil, scallion, asparagus and dill in a large skillet. Put from skillet over medium - high heat until asparagus is tender, around 10 minutes, then lift the mixture and set aside.

- •Sauté the salmon in the same skillet until flaky, about 10 minutes based on salmon thickness. Switch off skillet and set aside.

- •Wipe out the skillet on both sides with a paper towel and cook the eggs until lightly browned, about 5 minutes each side.

- •Put the salmon and asparagus mixture on half of the eggs, then turn the other half over to top. Serve.

DINNER

- •Grilled Shrimp and Black Bean Salad

This recipe is a perfect one to use while getting dinner service. No one knows this is low calorie!

Ingredients

•1 teaspoon of lime zest (approx. 1/2 lime)

•1/4 cup of freshly squeezed lime juice

•3 tablespoons of olive oil

•2 tablespoons of fresh basil chopped

•2 tablespoons of fresh oregano chopped

•1 teaspoon of freshly ground black pepper

•1/2 teaspoon of salt

•2 (15-ounce) cans of black beans, rinsed and washed

•1 cup of diced tomatoes

•1 cup of green bell pepper

•1/2 cup of chopped green onions

•24 large (21–25 count) raw shrimp, peeled and deveined

Preparation

•Combine lime zest and juice, olive oil, basil, oregano and pepper in a medium bowl, then mix well. Measure 2 tablespoons out and set aside in a small bowl.

•In a medium bowl, add the salt, black beans, tomatoes, bell pepper and onions and mix well. Put in fridge until served.

•Preheat the grill flat over medium to high heat. Place the shrimp on the rack until dry, and baste with the reserved lime juice mix. Cook on one side for 3 minutes then change, baste again and cook for another 3 minutes.

•Put a quarter of bean salad on each plate and top with 6 spicy shrimp to serve.

Day 3

BREAKFAST

•Old-Fashioned Sweet Potato Hash Browns

Not only are these sweet potato hash browns a great part of breakfast, they're also fantastic as a side for any dinner. When you make extra, when it's time to break your fast you will have them ready to go but you don't feel like eating.

Ingredients

•3 tablespoons coconut oil

•3 medium sweet potatoes, peeled and grated

•1 tablespoon ground cinnamon

Preparation

•Heat coconut oil over medium to high heat for 1 minute in a large sauté pan.

•Cook sweet potatoes over oil for 7 minutes, stirring frequently.

•Transfer potatoes, sprinkle with cinnamon and serve.

DINNER

•Mustard-Maple-Glazed Salmon

This is an incredibly delicious salmon recipe, especially given how simple and straightforward the preparation is. Add a baked sweet potato or some brown rice and have a sumptuous, flavourful meal.

Ingredients

•4 (6 ounces) skin-on salmon fillets, 3⁄4 inches thick

•1 teaspoon of olive oil

•1⁄2 teaspoon of salt

•1⁄2 teaspoon of freshly ground black pepper

•2 teaspoons of pure maple syrup

•½ teaspoon of dried mustard

•8 sprigs of fresh thyme

Preparation

•Preheat the grill flat over medium to high heat.

•Mix the salmon fillets with the olive oil on both sides, season with salt and pepper and put the skin side down on the grill. Cook them seven minutes.

•In the meantime, combine the maple syrup with dry mustard and a fork.

•Flip the salmon fillets, brush them with a maple-mustard glaze and top each with 2 thyme sprigs. Grill for another 5 to 7 minutes, or until the fish easily flakes.

•Use a spatula to transfer the fillets to 4 plates to serve, leaving the thyme intact.

Day 4

BREAKFAST

•Garlicky Vegetable-Packed Omelet

Delicious vegetables and garlic combine with fluffy eggs and white eggs to create a simple, satisfying and savory meal that starts right off any day! Protein-packed and rich in complex vegetable carbohydrates, this is a delicious way to get some nutritional value.

Ingredients

•Olive oil cooking spray

•¼ cup peeled and chopped yellow onion

•¼ cup sliced white mushrooms

•2 tablespoons filtered water

•2 teaspoons garlic powder

•¼ cup torn fresh spinach leaves

•3 large eggs

Preparation

•Paint a small frying pan with a spray of olive oil and steam over medium heat for 1 minute.

•Stir in onions and sauté for 1 minute. Add mushrooms and water and continue sautéing for about 4 minutes, until mushrooms are softened.

•Sprinkle onion-mushroom mixture with garlic powder and stir in the spinach leaves.

•Gather the eggs and pour over the sautéed vegetables the mixture of the eggs.

•Continue moving the outer edges of the mixture into the center right away for one turn around the whole tub. Let the omelet cook for 2 minutes untouched.

•Slide a spatula under an omelet, lifting it gently from the center of the pan. Once the omelet rests on the spatula, turn the omelet onto the other side easily.

•Continue to cook omelet for another 5 minutes until the omelet is pressed on and no juices remain. Fold over the eggs. Take it off heat and enjoy.

Gracious Garlic

A part of the lily flower family, garlic is a lovely plant that can lend your meal a seductive scent and unique taste. Use only one clove from this flexible plant's bulb to dress up bland dishes or add a savory new flavor.

DINNER

•Tuscan-Style Baked Sea

Bass Sea bass is a tasty fish—tasty and flaky. This Tuscan-inspired recipe supplements this mild fish with the flavors of fresh tomatoes, walnuts, basil, and garlic.

Ingredients

•4 (6-ounce) skin-on sea bass fillets

•1 teaspoon of olive oil

•1 cup of very finely chopped walnuts (use processor or blender)

•2 teaspoons of minced garlic

•8 slices of yellow or orange tomatoes, 1/4 inch thick

•8 slices of red onion, 1/4 inch thick

•1/2 cup of freshly chopped basil

•1/2 teaspoon of salt

•1/4 teaspoon of freshly ground black pepper

Preparation

•Preheat the oven to 400 degrees F, and line the aluminum foil baking sheet.

•Blend the olive oil on both sides of the bass fillets, then dip into the chopped walnuts, covering the filets completely. Place skin-side down the fillets onto the baking sheet. Layer the garlic over the fillets, and then coat the fish with alternating slices of tomato and onion. Sprinkle the basil over the top and salt and pepper to season.

•Bake for 12-14 minutes, or quickly until the fish flakes. Use a spatula to move the filets onto 4 plates to serve.

Day 5

BREAKFAST

•Very Vegetable Frittata

Packed with plenty of egg white and yolk protein and rich in carbs from all the fresh vegetables, this sumptuous frittata will leave you complete and energized. Use your favorite veggies to customize!

Ingredients

•Olive oil cooking spray

•½ cup chopped fresh broccoli florets

•½ cup diced white mushrooms

•½ cup seeded and chopped yellow bell pepper

•¼ yellow onion, peeled and finely chopped

•¼ cup filtered water

•8 large eggs

•1 tablespoon garlic powder

•1 teaspoon sea salt

•2 teaspoons freshly ground black pepper

Preparation

•Preheat oven to 350 degrees F. Grease a big, oven-safe skillet with a spray of olive oil and preheat for 1 minute over medium heat.

•In a pan, mix broccoli, mushrooms, bell pepper and onions with water and cook for about 5 minutes, until tender but not heavy.

•Whisk the eggs, garlic powder, salt and black pepper together and scatter over the vegetables.

•Fry before mixing center begins trembling and heat bubbling, about 4 minutes.

•Remove the skillet from the heat and put it in a preheated
oven for 15 minutes until the mixture center is fixed and
the fork inserted is clean. Cut, and serve in wedges.

DINNER

•Flank Steak Spinach Salad

Flank steak is a light and tasty beef cut suitable for a low-
calorie diet. This recette includes medium-rare cooking of the
steak. When cooked much more than that, the meat seems to
get rather lean.

Ingredients

•1 pound steak, visible fat and sinew extracted

•1⁄4 cup Balsamic Vinaigrette (see Avocado and Fennel
Salad with Balsamic Vinaigrette for directions)

•1⁄2 teaspoon salt

•1⁄2 teaspoon of freshly ground black pepper

•3 cups of sliced roman lettuce

•1 cup of baby spinach leaves.

•1-pint cherry tomatoes halved

•½ cup thinly sliced sweet yellow onion

Preparation

•Preheat the grill flat over high heat until dry.

•Spray the steak on the flank with 2 Balsamic Vinaigrette spoonfuls, season with salt and pepper and put on the grill. Cook for 5 minutes, then turn over and cook for another 10 minutes or until medium-rare steak is available.

•In the meantime, add the spinach, cabbage, tomatoes and onion until well combined. Then add the 2 teaspoons of vinaigrette dressing left over. I toss to coat and split the salad into 4 bowls.

•Move the flank steak to the plate and require it to sit on the diagonal for 10 minutes before slicing thinly.

•Put 1/4 of the sliced steak on top of each salad and serve

Day6

BREAKFAST

•Heavenly Hash Browns

In this excellent hash browns recipe, the classic version of this favorite breakfast gets a complete overhaul. You will indulge every last taste of these tasty hash browns by using good, fresh ingredients and swapping the not - so-healthy oils with a small quantity of olive oil.

Ingredients

•Olive oil cooking spray

•3 medium Idaho potatoes, scrubbed and shredded

•1 small yellow onion, peeled and minced

•1 large egg

•1 teaspoon garlic powder

•¼ teaspoon sea salt

•¼ teaspoon freshly ground black pepper

•1 tablespoon olive oil

Preparation

•Fill a large skillet with a spray of olive oil and preheat for 1 minute over medium heat.

•Combine shredded potatoes, onions, egg and garlic powder in a large mixing bowl and stir until thoroughly mixed. Season with salt and pepper.

•Shape potato mixture into thick patties using ½ cup of each patty mixture.

•In a pan, heat olive oil for 1 minute and add two brown hashed patties. Cook until golden brown, for 5 minutes.

•Flip the patties and continue cooking for another 4 minutes until both sides are golden brown and fully cooked through. Replace cycle with remaining patties and repeat process.

DINNER

•Easy Black Bean Soup

This dish is a comforting and filling meal, when served with a fresh salad and a crusty roll. You will get all the typical black bean soup flavors, but in far less time.

Ingredients

•2 (15-ounce) cans black beans

•½ teaspoon chili powder

•2 cups chicken stock

•1 cup thinly sliced carrots

•½ cup chopped yellow onion

•½ teaspoon garlic powder

•½ teaspoon ground cumin

•½ teaspoon salt

•¼ teaspoon freshly ground black pepper

•1 cup plain yoghurt

•¼ cup sliced green onions

Preparation

•Mix the black beans, chicken stock, carrots, onion, garlic powder, cumin, chili powder and salt in a large saucepan over medium to high heat. Shake good.

•Bring the soup to a boil, reduce the heat to mild, cover and simmer, stirring occasionally for 20 minutes.

•Finish with a big dollop of cream, ladle in 4 bowls and garnish with green onions.

Day 7

BREAKFAST

•Pumpkin Spice Smoothie

If you are looking for a break from the regular fruit smoothie, mix your things in a bowl with this tasty pumpkin pie! Raw ingredients and spicy spices make this organic smoothie one of the healthiest and most delicious breakfast choices available.

Ingredients

•1 cup canned sweet potato purée

•1 cup unsweetened vanilla almond milk

•1 teaspoon ground cloves

•1 teaspoon ground ginger

•1 teaspoon ground cinnamon

•24 ice cubes (approximately 2 cups)

Preparation

•In a blender, add sweet potato purée, sugar, and spices with half ice and blend until well mixed.

•Gradually add the remaining ice and combine until desired.

DINNER

•Hearty Vegetable Soup

This soup is easy to make and has a wide range of vegetables. It's a great soup for those days when you don't feel like eating to serve alongside a salad or sandwich so double up and freeze the extra.

Ingredients

•1 teaspoon of olive oil

•1 cup of Yukon Gold potatoes

•1/2 cup of thinly sliced carrots

•1⁄2 cup of fresh green beans, cut into 1-inch pieces

•1⁄2 cup of chopped yellow onion

•1 cup of fresh spinach leaves

•3 cups of chicken stock

•1⁄4 cup of fresh chopped parsley

•1⁄2 cup of chopped fresh rosemary

•1⁄2 cup of salt

•1⁄4 cup of freshly ground black pepper

Preparation

•Heat the olive oil in a large, heavy skillet over medium - high heat. Remove the cabbage, carrots, green beans and onion and sauté, stirring frequently for 5 minutes. Out of heat remove.

•Move the vegetables over medium-high heat to a large saucepan. Stir in spinach, chicken stock, parsley, rosemary, salt and pepper and bring to a boil the soup. Reduce heat to medium, cover for 30 minutes and simmer.

Day 8

BREAKFAST

- Huevos Rancheros Without Tortillas

This is a classic Southern Border dish. If you eat grains, brown rice tortillas can be used to turn these into burritos for breakfast.

Ingredients

- 3 tablespoons olive oil, divided

- 2 medium vine-ripened tomatoes, finely chopped

- 2 small shallots, finely chopped

- ½ teaspoon sea salt, divided

- 2 large eggs

- ¼ teaspoon freshly ground pepper

- ¼ cup fresh cilantro leaves

•1 medium jalapeño pepper, stemmed, seeded, and finely chopped

Preparation

•In a non-stick oven, heat 2 spoons of oil over medium heat for 1 minute.

•Add the tomatoes and shallots to the pan and ¼ teaspoon salt to season. Cover the pan and let cook, occasionally stirring for about 5 minutes until shallots are limp. Set aside the blend.

•Heat the remaining tablespoon of oil over medium heat for 1 minute in medium non-stick skillet.

•Break eggs into skillet and cook sunny until white and yolks are fluffy, around 2 minutes. If you prefer fully cooked yolks, cook the eggs with skillet covered for an additional minute.

•Put each egg on a plate. Pour the tomato mixture onto the shells, completely covering every shell.

•Season the remaining salt and pepper with the eggs and garnish with half cilantro and jalapeño for each egg.

Top It Off with an Avocado

Consider your Huevos Rancheros a full meal, with half a sliced avocado served on top of each sandwich. Avocados are a rich source of healthy fats: they are made up of 67 per cent monosaturated fats that support cardiovascular health.

DINNER

•Tapenade with feta

The paste of olive can taste excessively strong and sharp, but it does make a tangy and creamy spread in combination with the feta. Delicious on coin-shaped courgette slices as canapés or spread on seed crackers – or just eaten as a dip.

Calorie content: 138 calories

Ingredients

•50g feta 50g pitted olives, from a jar or tin, drained

•1 tablespoon of olive oil

Preparation

•Mix the ingredients in a small bowl with a handheld blender, leaving some chunky bits of olive oil.

Day 9

BREAKFAST

•Farmers' Scrambler

Farmers understand a healthy breakfast is the best way to prepare for long working days. Starting your rough day will allow you to complete it solid.

Ingredients

•2 cups peeled and diced Russet potatoes

•3 tablespoons olive oil, divided

•½ cup sliced white mushrooms

•¼ cup seeded and chopped red bell peppers

•¼ cup peeled and chopped red onion

•8 large eggs

•¼ teaspoon salt

•¼ teaspoon freshly ground black pepper

Preparation

•In a medium sauté pan, sauté potatoes over medium heat in 1½ tablespoons of olive oil until soft, about 10 minutes.

•Heat the remaining oil in a small medium sauce pan, add the mushrooms, peppers and onions and sauté over medium heat for 5 minutes.

•In one large pan, add the contents of both panes.

•Crack eggs in a medium sized dish. Add to vegetable mixture and scramble for 3 minutes over medium heat.

•Season with salt and pepper to taste.

Give It a French Touch

To give your scrambler something special, add 1 tablespoon of the classic French herb blend herbes de Provence. Typically this combination includes savory marjoram, rosemary, thyme, oregano and lavender. This herbal mix can be sold in most supermarkets.

DINNER

•Marinated London Broil

When it comes to steak rubs, cinnamon and cloves may not be your first idea, but these spices deliver mouthwatering flavors. Split the London broil off the grain after cooking.

Ingredients

•1 cup dry red wine

•1 tablespoon olive oil

•1 teaspoon ground cinnamon

•½ teaspoon ground cloves

•1 teaspoon ground cumin

•¼ teaspoon freshly cracked black peppercorns

•¼ teaspoon salt

•1½ pounds London broil

Preparation

•Preheat to medium-heat grill.

•Blend the juice, the oil and seasonings together. Coat in a mixture of meat, then grill to desired doneness. Chop and drink.

Day 10

BREAKFAST

•Low Fat Mini-Quiche

Ingredients

•4 eggs (OR for less fat-1 cup of a plain egg substitute, such as "Egg Beaters")

•1⁄2 cup cookie mix, such as Bisquick

•1/3 cup Melted butter

•11⁄2 cup Milk skim

•Pepper

•1 TBS. Flakes of onion or 2 tsp. Onion powder

•4 ounces of low-fat shredded cheddar cheese• Sliced mushrooms and / or steamed asparagus (optional)

Preparation

•Place everything in the blender except cheese and optional
vegetables until smooth, add vegetables and stir to mix
in, put into an oil-sprinkled mini-muffin tray, cover
with shredded cheese, bake at 350 degrees for 30
minutes (or until eggs are set). Let sit in a tray to cool
for 15-20 minutes before removing. These can be frozen
individually on a greased cookie sheet, and placed in a
zipper freezer bag once frozen. Attach and microwave
what you need for a perfect make-ahead mini-breakfast
for 30 seconds (or more-ovens vary).

DINNER

•Smoky Black-Eyed Pea Soup with Sweet Potatoes and
Mustard Greens

Black-eyed peas offer green peas with a delicious earthiness
but with a savory touch. Use any dark, fresh or frozen leafy
greens you'd like, instead of the mustard greens. Julienned
kale or collard greens are great choices and are high in
antioxidants as well.

Ingredients

•1 tablespoon olive oil

•1 medium yellow onion, peeled and chopped

•2 stalks celery, chopped

•1 large carrot, peeled and chopped

•2 teaspoons salt

•1 teaspoon dried thyme

•2 teaspoons dried oregano

•1 teaspoon ground cumin

•1 dried chipotle chili, halved

•2 bay leaves

•1 pound dried black-eyed peas, washed and picked through for undesirables

•2 quarts vegetable stock

•1 large sweet potato, peeled and diced into 1' cubes

•1 (10-ounce) package frozen mustard greens, chopped

•1 (22-ounce) can diced tomatoes, drained

•¼ teaspoon chopped fresh cilantro

Preparation

•Heat the oil 1 minute over medium heat in a big, heavy-bottomed Dutch oven. Add onion, celery, carrot and salt and simmer for 5 minutes until translucent. Add thyme, oregano, cumin, chipotle chili and bay leaves; add 2 minutes to cook.

•Remove the vegetable stock and the black-eyed peas. Bring to a boil on high heat, then cook for 2 hours on low heat until the beans are very tender.

•Pour in the sweet potato and roast for 20 minutes. Add chopped mustard and tomatoes. Cook for another 10 minutes, until the potatoes and greens are soft. Change consistency with supplementary vegetable stock. The soup should contain plenty of broth.

•Garnished with chopped coriander.

Day 11

BREAKFAST

•Low-Fat Banana Bread:

Ingredients

•3 Cups of all-purpose flour (or 2 white cups and 1 whole wheat cup)

•1½ Cups of sugar

•2½ tsp. Baking powder

•1 tablespoon Soda Baking

•1 tsp. Cinnamon

•4 egg whites

•4 medium or 3 bigger mashed bananas

•1/2 cup of unsweetened applesauce

Preparation

•Mix the egg whites with the bananas and applesauce in one dish.

•Pour the flour, sugar, salt, soda and cinnamon into another larger bowl.

•In a dry bowl, add the wet bowl and stir until just mixed. Use TBS if heavy. Hot water

•Spoon flour into an 8 inch X 4 inch greased bread pan and bake at 350 degrees for 45-55 minutes. Cool, on a rack of wire.

DINNER

•Lentil Soup with Cumin

This is the best bean soup you can get ready in an hour. This gets better as it sits overnight so make enough for two or more meals when the flavors meet!

Ingredients

•½ teaspoon whole cumin seeds

•1 tablespoon olive oil

•1 large carrot, peeled and chopped

•1 stalk celery, chopped

•1 medium yellow onion, peeled and chopped

•1 large Russet potato, peeled and chopped

•2 cloves garlic, peeled and sliced

•2 teaspoons salt

•1 cup dried lentils

•2 quarts vegetable stock

Preparation

•In a dry, dry saucepan, toast cumin seeds for 1 minute until fragrant.

•Heat the oil in a large pot over medium heat for 1 minute. Attach the onions, cumin, garlic, and butter. Cook on for 5 minutes.

•Add the vegetable stock and lentils. To bring soup to a boil, raise heat to high, then decrease heat to medium-low. Simmer on for 1 hour.

•Serve warm.

Day 12

BREAKFAST

•Super Easy Pasta Salad

Ingredients

•1 pkg. bow-tie pasta (16 ounce)

•2 sliced cucumbers

•6 chopped tomatoes

•1 bunch of chopped green onions

•4 ounces of grated Parmesan cheese

•1 TBS. Seasoning Italian

Preparation

•Cook pasta for al dente, drain and rinse under cold water according to instructions–then place in a large tub. Toss the vegetables and pasta and the salad dressing together. Mix the parmesan cheese and Italian seasoning in a separate small pot, then insert softly into pasta salad. Cover and leave to cool. Makes eight cups. Good idea for a dinner with your mates.

DINNER

•Tuscan White Bean Soup

Beans are full of fiber, not only keeping you regular but keeping you full longer. This tasty White Bean Soup from Tuscany will keep the appetite at place.

Ingredients

•2 tablespoons extra-virgin olive oil, divided

•1 medium yellow onion, peeled and chopped

•1 large leek, white part only, finely chopped

•3 cloves garlic, peeled and finely chopped

•3 teaspoons fresh chopped rosemary

•1 bay leaf

•3 quarts vegetable stock

•2 cups large white beans (soaked overnight if desired)

•1/4 teaspoon salt

•1/4 teaspoon ground white pepper

Preparation

•Heat 1 tablespoon of olive oil for 1 minute in a large medium heat soup pot. Add onion, leeks, and garlic; cook for 10 minutes until translucent, frequently stirring onions. Add the rosemary and bay leaf, and cook for another 5 minutes.

•Apply potted stock and beans. Take to a full hot boil. Reduce heat to low and cook for 90 minutes until the very tender beans begin to fall apart. Cooking time for soaked beans can vary depending on the age of the

beans and whether or not they have been soaked;
expect 30 minutes less.

•Puree 2/3 soup in mixer; add back to soup remainder.
Season with pepper and salt.

•Serve each bowl sprinkled with a couple of drops of extra
virgin olive oil.

Soaking Beans—What It Means

Some chefs submerge beans overnight in water before frying.
In much less time the beans swell with water and cook.
However soaked beans appear to break up more than
unsoaked ones, so cooking beans from a dry state can be
helpful.

Day 13

BREAKFAST

•Low-fat Oven-Baked Chicken Nuggets

Ingredients

•3 skinless, boneless chicken breasts, cut into strips

•1 cup Italian-flavored Bread Crumbs

•½ cup low-fat Parmesan cheese

•1 tsp. Salt

•1 tsp (optional) Thyme

•1 dc. 1 Egg white basil

•¼ cup skim milk

Preparation

•Heat the oven to 400 degrees, put an oven-proof greased cooling rack on top of a cookie sheet (or grate the cookie sheet and bypass the cooling rack–the cooling rack keeps it crispy on all sides!).

•Combine the bread crumbs, seasonings, cheese and salt in one small large bowl; whisk the egg white and the milk together in another small bowl.

•Dunk the strips of chicken into the mixture of egg / milk– then into the mixture of bread crumbs to cover on all sides. Place the strips on the refrigerated rack (or directly on the cookie sheet).

•Bake for 20 minutes

•Freeze on a greased cookie sheet-put nuggets in a zipper bag when frozen and just pull out what you need. For three strips, heat up in microwave for 40 seconds (oven times may vary).

DINNER

•Vegan Chili

Through frying the beef with the onions, you can add some ground beef or ground turkey to this recipe, whether you want a meaty chili. This hearty chili will keep you full (and satisfied!) for hours, with or without the beef.

Ingredients

- ¼ cup olive oil

- 2 cups peeled and chopped yellow onion

- 1 cup peeled and chopped carrots

- 2 cups chopped and seeded assorted bell peppers

- 2 teaspoons salt

- 4 teaspoons ground cumin

- 1 tablespoon peeled and chopped garlic

- 2 medium jalapeño peppers, stemmed, seeded, and chopped

•1 tablespoon ground ancho chili pepper

•1 chipotle in adobo, chopped

•1 (28-ounce) can plum tomatoes, roughly chopped, juice
included

•3 (15.5-ounce) cans beans: 1 red kidney, 1 cannellini, and 1
black, drained and rinsed

•1 cup tomato juice

•2 tablespoons peeled and finely chopped red onions

•2 tablespoons chopped fresh cilantro

Preparation

•Heat oil over medium heat for 1 minute in a big, heavy-
bottomed Dutch oven or soup pot. Remove onions,
carrots, bell peppers, and salt; simmer over medium
heat for 15 minutes, until the ointments are smooth.

•Toast the cumin 1 minute in a hot, dry skillet over medium heat. In Dutch oven, add garlic, jalapeños, ancho and chipotle; cook another 5 minutes.

•Apply onions, beans and tomato juice to compare. Simmer had covered at low heat for 45 minutes.

•Serve garnished with cilantro and red onions.

Day 14

BREAKFAST

•Pumpkin Oatmeal

Ingredients

•½ cup steel cut oats

•1 cup water

•1/3 cup pumpkin (canned pumpkin)

•½ cup skim milk (cow, goat, rice milk or soy milk)

•1 tsp vanilla

•1 dash cinnamon

•1 dash nutmeg

•t tbs raw walnuts and almonds (crushed or slivered)

•1 tsp maple syrup

Preparation

•Add oats and water to a 2 quarter sauce pan

•Bring to a boil, stirring occasionally

•Lower to simmer

•Cook until fluffy for around 8-10 minutes

•Add milk

•Add pumpkin

•Add ginger, nutmeg and cinnamon

•Add nuts and or maple syrup.

DINNER

•Zucchini "Lasagna"

This wheat-free casserole is best made a day in advance, layered and baked like the beloved Italian-American pasta dish. If you don't have a mandolin or slicing machine, your store's deli-counter may be happy to slice your zucchini out.

Ingredients

- •3 cups tomato sauce, divided

- •4 large zucchini, sliced lengthwise about 1/8' thick, divided

- •¼ teaspoon salt

- •¼ teaspoon freshly ground black pepper

- •1 pound ricotta cheese, divided

- •1 pound shredded mozzarella cheese, divided

- •2 cups frozen mixed vegetables, thawed, divided

Preparation

•Preheat oven to 350 degrees F.

•Press 1 cup of tomato sauce on the bottom of a baking dish of 9' or 13.' Arrange a sheet of slices of zucchini in the pan, with slightly overlapping slices.

•Dot layer of zucchini with half of ricotta, spreading teaspoonful evenly around the casserole. Layer a third of shredded cheese over ricotta, then half of thawed vegetables over layer.

•Arrange another sheet of zucchini and replicate the fillings with the remaining ricotta, remaining vegetables and another portion of the shredded cheese; Remove the final layer of zucchini and scatter over the remaining tomato sauce.

•Sprinkle over with remaining cheese; bake for 1 hour until the saucepan is bubbled and the cheese is slightly brown. Slightly cool down, about 10 minutes before cutting and serving.

Zucchini Lasagna Twist

Try to replace half the zucchini with an equal portion of an eggplant in this recipe. Be sure to use small, smooth strips, which are dusted very gently with salt on one side.

Day 15

BREAKFAST

•Banana Split Oatmeal

Ingredients

•1/3 cup oatmeal, quick-cooking (dry)

•1/8 teaspoon salt

•¾ cups water (very hot)

•½ banana (sliced)

•½ cup frozen yogurt, non-fat

Preparation

•Blend the oatmeal and the salt together in a microwave
protected cereal bowl. Stir the water back.

•Microwave for 1 minute on high-power. Cut. Microwave another minute on high power. Stir up.

•Microwave on high power for another 30-60 seconds until the cereal reaches the desired thickness. Stir again.

•Complete with sliced bananas and frozen yogurt.

DINNER

•Chicken Lettuce Cups

These Chicken Lettuce Cups make a great light meal, easy to whip up and easy to eat, too. Whether you integrate grains into your fasting routine, you can enjoy these cups on your own or match them with a side of brown rice.

Ingredients

•3 pounds ground chicken

•1/8 teaspoon finely chopped fresh gingerroot

•2 (8-ounce) cans water chestnuts, drained and chopped

•¼ cup chili powder

•2 tablespoons coconut oil

•½ cup coconut aminos

•2 tablespoons rice wine vinegar

•½ cup chopped scallions, green parts only

•1 tablespoon freshly squeezed lime juice

•16 large inner leaves of iceberg lettuce, trimmed and chilled

Preparation

•Add the chicken, ginger, water chestnuts, and chili powder in a large bowl. Combine both hands well.

•Heat the oil over medium heat in a large skillet for 1 minute. Apply mixture to the chicken. For carve chicken into small chunks use a spatula. Stir in aminos, sugar, scallions, and lime juice; simmer for 8 minutes until chicken is cooked.

•Arrange leaves of lettuce over a plate and fill each leaf with a mixture of 1/4 cup meat. Wrap the lettuce into a blend. Serve straightaway.

Day 16

BREAKFAST

•Healthy Breakfast Frittata

Ingredients

•½ medium onion, minced

•4 medium cloves garlic, chopped

•1/4 lb. ground lamb or turkey

•1 + 2 tbs chicken broth

•3 cups rinsed and finely chopped kale (stems removed)

•5 omega-3 enriched eggs

•Salt and black pepper to taste

Preparation

•Slim the onion and cut the garlic; require them to sit for 5
minutes to improve their health benefits.

•Preheat broiler on low.

•Warm a 9-10 inch stainless steel skillet with 1 TBS broth.
Sauté the onion over medium heat, stirring regularly,
for about 3 minutes.

•Add the garlic, lamb or turkey and cook over medium heat
for another 3 minutes, breaking up clumps.

•Add the kale and the broth 2 TBS. Reduce heat to low, and
keep cooking covered for about 5 minutes longer.
Season with salt and pepper, then pour water.

•Mix whites, season with a pinch of salt and pepper and
scatter thinly on top of mixture. Cook on medium,
without stirring for another 2 minutes.

•Put skillet in the center of the oven under the broiler,
about 7 inches from the heat source, so you have time to
cook without the top burning. It is over, about 2-3
minutes after the eggs are solid.

DINNER

•Slow Cooker Chicken Tagine

Tagine is a stew from Morocco, and is used in many parts of North Africa as well. In Cypriot cuisine it is also known as tavas. Try this simpler version of a more conventional tagine recipe.

Ingredients

•1½ tablespoons sweet paprika

•1 teaspoon ground cinnamon

•1½ tablespoons ground coriander

•1½ teaspoons ground turmeric

•2 teaspoons ground cardamom

•1½ teaspoons ground allspice

•1/8 teaspoon wheat-free asafetida powder

•¼ teaspoon sea salt

•¼ teaspoon freshly ground black pepper

•4 (5-ounce) skinless, boneless chicken thighs, halved

•1 tablespoon olive oil

•1½ teaspoons ground ginger

•1½ teaspoons saffron

•1 (14-ounce) can whole tomatoes, drained

•1/3 cup canned chickpeas, thoroughly drained and rinsed

•1 quart chicken stock

•1 lemon, chopped into wedges

•1 tablespoon chopped fresh flat-leaf parsley

Preparation

•In a small pan, toast paprika, cinnamon, coriander, turmeric, cardamom and allspice for about 2 minutes, until it is fragrant. Set aside, and require 3 minutes to cool.

•Once cooled, sprinkle each half-thigh chicken with spice mixture, asafetida, salt and pepper on both sides.

•Heat the oil over medium heat in a large skillet for 1 minute. Add the chicken thighs and sear until browned, on each side for about 2 minutes. Remove the chicken from heat and place in a 4–6-quarter slow cooker.

•Include ginger in skillet. Cook for 2 minutes, then stir.

•To slow cooker, add the ginger, saffron, onions, chickpeas, and chicken stock. Cook for 4 hours on fast. Once finished, remove to serve with lemon and parsley and garnish with dish.

Day 17

BREAKFAST

•Crustless Spinach Pie

Ingredients

•2 tablespoons butter

•2 eggs (large)

•½ cup flour

•½ cup milk (1%)

•2 garlic cloves (minced, or 1/2 teaspoon garlic powder)

•½ teaspoon baking powder

•4 ounces mozzarella

•2 cups spinach (chopped, fresh)

Preparation

•Preheat oven to 350 ° C.

•Melt butter or margarine in an 8 "baking saucepan.

•Whisk eggs well. Add flour, baking powder, milk and garlic. Pour into a pan to bake. Stir in spinach and cheese.

•Bake for 30-35 minutes or until the cheese is golden brown and solid.

DINNER

•Fish Curry

The salmon in this Fish Curry contains a healthy dose of omega-3 fatty acids that can help you combat depression and maintain healthy brain conditions.

Ingredients

•1 medium carrot, peeled and chopped

•2 cups chicken broth

•¼ teaspoon gluten-free fish sauce

•1 (13.5-ounce) can unsweetened full-fat coconut milk, refrigerated overnight, cream only

•1 medium Roma or vine-ripe tomato, diced

•½ small stalk celery, diced

•1 tablespoon curry powder

•¼ teaspoon ground cumin

•¼ teaspoon ground coriander

•½ teaspoon ground turmeric

•¼ teaspoon freshly grated ginger

•2 tablespoons roughly chopped fresh cilantro

•½ pound wild-caught salmon, skin removed

Preparation

•Boil the carrots over high heat in a medium saucepan until only slightly hardened, around 3 minutes. Drain, recycle water, then whisk in chicken broth and fish sauce.

•Apply banana, onion, celery, curry powder, cumin, cilantro and turmeric to the saucepan.

•Cover,. heat to low and simmer for 20 minutes, stirring every 5 minutes;

•Blend with cilantro and ginger. Add the fish and stir in liquid to cover.

•Cook over medium heat for 5 minutes to produce flaccid shrimp, and then serve.

Day 18

BREAKFAST

•Greek Yogurt Parfait

Ingredients

•3 cups plain fat-free Greek-style yogurt (such as Fage)

•1 teaspoon vanilla extract

•4 teaspoons honey

•28 clementine segments

•¼ cup shelled, unsalted dry-roasted chopped pistachios

Preparation

•Mix vanilla and milk in a tub. Spoon 1/3 cup yogurt mixture into each of 4 thin, beautiful glasses; top with

½ teaspoon honey, 5 pieces of clementine and ½ tablespoon nuts each.

•Top parfaits with the remaining yogurt mixture (approximately 1/3 cup each); finish with ½ teaspoon sugar, 2 slices of clementine and ½ tablespoon almonds. Serve straightaway.

DINNER

•Filet Mignon Salad

In this filling salad, filet mignon, the tenderness and most popular beef cut, is dressed to the nines in greens, tomatoes and goat cheese.

Ingredients

•¼ large head romaine lettuce, chopped and ribs removed

•½ large head Belgian endive (about 11/2cups), trimmed and thinly sliced crosswise

•¼ cup chopped fresh basil

•1½ cups baby arugula

•2 teaspoons pure maple syrup

•½ cup rice wine vinegar

•1½ tablespoons freshly squeezed lemon juice

•½ teaspoon sea salt

•½ teaspoon freshly ground black pepper

•½ cup plus 1½ teaspoons olive oil, divided

•1 tablespoon unsalted grass-fed butter

•½ pound filet mignon

•2 ounces crumbled goat cheese

•8 cherry tomatoes, halved

Preparation

•Mix the romaine, endive, basil, and arugula in a large salad bowl.

•Add the maple syrup, vinegar, lemon juice, salt and pepper to a food processor or blender. With the machine running at low velocity, slowly pour in ½ cup gasoline. Deposit back.

•Melt butter in a small cast iron skillet or stainless steel skillet with remaining olive oil over medium heat for 1 minute. Add mignon filet and cook for medium-rare (or longer, depending on the ideal degree of doneness) for 7 minutes each side. Remove from heat and let stand for 5 minutes. Slice into fairly thick strips.

•Add salad bowl of mignon filet, goat cheese and cherry tomatoes. Pour the sheets back. Toss to coat well and then drink.

Day 19

BREAKFAST

•Barley with Banana & Sunflower Seeds

Ingredients

•2/3 cup water

•1/3 cup uncooked quick-cooking pearl barley

•1 banana, sliced

•1 tablespoon unsalted salted sunflower seeds

•1 teaspoon honey

Preparation

•In a small microwave-safe bowl, combine 2/3 cup water and the barley. Microwave 6 minutes on Max.

•Stir 2 minutes and let rise.

•Complete with banana slices, honey and sunflower seeds.

DINNER

•Zoodles with Pesto

It's not just fun to make "zoodles," or zucchini noodles, but also a nutritious way to enjoy pasta dishes.

Ingredients

•¾ cup fresh basil leaves

•2 tablespoons garlic-infused olive oil

•¼ cup pine nuts

•2 tablespoons extra-virgin olive oil

•½ cup freshly grated Parmesan cheese

•¼ teaspoon sea salt, divided

- ¼ teaspoon freshly ground black pepper, divided

- 1 tablespoon olive oil

- 1 pound zucchini, peeled into long, narrow ribbons

Preparation

- Mix the basil, garlic oil and pine nuts in a food processor for pesto sauce and pulse until strongly chopped. Attach the olive oil, cheese, 1/8 teaspoon salt and 1/8 teaspoon pepper and smoothly process.

- Heat the olive oil 1 minute over medium heat in a medium sauté pan. Add the zucchini noodles, 1/8 teaspoon salt and 1/8 teaspoon pepper to the pan and stir for 5 minutes until tender. Serve with a sauce made with pesto.

Flavored Oils

Store herbs, spices and garlic cloves in a bottle of oil and steep for at least three days or up to two weeks to infuse oil with flavor and complexity. When scented with rosemary, thyme, savory, garlic, peppercorns, dried mushrooms, or truffles, fine olive oil becomes a transcendent condiment. Infused oils can also be bought at gourmet stores.

Day 20

BREAKFAST

•Chinese Chicken Cabbage Salad

Ingredients

•4 cups napa cabbage, sliced thin

•1 TBS extra virgin olive oil

•1 TBS rice vinegar

•1 tsp soy sauce

•1 TBS minced ginger

•1 medium clove garlic, pressed

•2 TBS chopped cilantro

•4 oz cooked chicken breast, shredded or cut into 1″ cubes

Preparation

Toss all ingredients together and serve.

DINNER

•Chicken Burgers

This basic recipe becomes a favorite for your sporadic period of fasting. Chicken Burgers are easy to whip up and are well stored so you can have a quick meal on the go. You can also make them your own by adding meat and spices of any sort.

Ingredients

•1 pound ground chicken

•½ teaspoon salt

•½ teaspoon ground white pepper

•1 large egg, beaten

•¼ cup grated Parmesan cheese

•1 tablespoon olive oil

Preparation

•Combine all ingredients, except oil, with your hands in a large bowl until well blended.

•Turn the mixture into 4 patties.

•Heat the oil over medium - high 1 minute in a large skillet and add burgers. Cook about 5 minutes on one side, then turn over and cook on the other side, about 5 minutes before cooked through.

Day 21

BREAKFAST

•Mediterranean Tabouli Salad

Ingredients

•1 cup wheat bulgur (dry), makes 2 cups after combining
   with liquid

•½ medium onion, minced

•2 cloves garlic, pressed or chopped

•3 cups minced fresh parsley

•1 medium tomato, chopped

•3 tbs extra virgin olive oil

•1 tbs fresh lemon juice or wine vinegar

•Sea salt and pepper to taste

Preparation

•Place 1 cup of bulgur wheat and salt into a bowl to taste. Pour 2 cups of boiling water or broth over the bulgur, stir once and let sit until liquid is absorbed for 15-20 minutes.

•Squeeze the onion and pinch or cut the garlic and let it rest for 5 minutes to bring out its secret property.

•Put all the ingredients together and put properly.

•You might want to add more olive oil and lemon juice for added flavor.

DINNER

•Pork and Fennel Meatballs

Those meatballs can be described as earthy and certainly delicious. Serve either as an appetizer or as a full meal with a sprinkle of chopped fresh parsley, with pasta and marinara sauce.

Ingredients

- •1 pound 84 percent lean ground pork

- •2 tablespoons roughly chopped fresh flat-leaf parsley

- •3 tablespoons almond meal

- •1 large egg

- •¼ teaspoon salt

- •½ teaspoon freshly ground black pepper

- •1½ tablespoons olive oil

- •2 teaspoons fennel seeds

Preparation

- •Mix the bacon, parsley, coconut, potato, salt, and pepper in a mixing bowl. Form the blend into 24 (1') meatballs.

•Heat oil over medium heat for 1 minute in a medium skillet and sauté fennel seeds for about 4 minutes, until they are fragrant.

•Blend in meatballs. Brown meatballs on all sides, for a total of about 20 minutes. Meatballs are fried internally, when they are no longer pink.

Problems to Watch For

For anyone with a health condition but especially for diabetics, close monitoring during fasting is essential. If you are taking insulin, you should monitor blood sugar at least four times daily. If you feel any hypoglycemic symptoms, such as shaking or sweating, you should check your blood sugar immediately.

The blood pressure is to be regularly monitored. With any of the widely available apps, that can be done at home. Make sure to talk with your doctor about daily blood work like electrolyte assessment. We often monitor the calcium, phosphorus, and magnesium levels in addition to the usual electrolytes.

If you feel unwell for whatever reason, immediately stop fasting and see your doctor. In fact, recurrent nausea, vomiting, dizziness, fatigue, high or low sugar in the blood and lethargy with sporadic or prolonged fasting are not common and should raise a red flag.

Nevertheless, hunger and constipation are common symptoms, and can be controlled.

Feasts and Fasts: Understanding the Rhythms of Life

Family and friends celebrations form an integral part of a well lived life. We need to remind ourselves every once in a while that life is sweet and we're lucky to be alive. And we've done that throughout human history, through feasting. The very act of eating is a celebration of life, and we do so with a feast when we are celebrating important events. Any diet not knowing the reality is doomed to failure. We eat birthday cake. They have seasonal feasts, such as Thanksgiving and Christmas. We plan banquets for wedding parties. On the day of our wedding we go to a nice restaurant.

We don't celebrate with salad for birthday. We don't eat the replacement bars for wedding meals. On Thanksgiving we don't gorge on the green shakes.

Like all of life, weight gain isn't constant; it's sporadic. Many lifetimes are correlated with heightened weight gain. It includes puberty, where weight gain is part of normal growth, and abortion, where weight gain is common and necessary.

The rest of the weight gain of the year comes around the holidays in a short period of time each year. The period from

Thanksgiving to New Year's only covers six weeks but it accounts for about two-thirds of the 1.4-pound (on average) weight gain in the year.

If weight gain isn't consistent throughout the year, then weight loss efforts also need to vary. You need a technique that at some times promotes weight loss and at other times holds on weight. A constant diet reduced in calories does not match the feast and fast cycle, and is therefore doomed to failure.

There are days you'd have to eat a lot. Some days you should eat just about nothing. That is the natural life cycle. This is known by most major religions by offering feasts at certain times — for example, Christmas— and fasting at others, such as the Lent. The ancient civilizations understood the basic rhythm of life as well. They had been feasting when the harvest came in. But, in winter, they often fasted.

The Dawn Phenomenon

For those not acquainted with the Dawn Phenomenon, the phenomenon of high blood sugar after a time of fasting is often puzzling. Why are blood sugars high, if you haven't been eating for a while? Even with prolonged fasting that effect is seen.

The Dawn Phenomenon, also referred to as the Dawn Effect, was first identified some 30 years ago. It is estimated to occur in diabetics of type 2 up to 75 percent, although severity varies widely, and is caused by circadian rhythms.

The body secretes higher levels of growth hormone, cortisol, glucagon and adrenaline just before awakening (around 4:00 a.m.). Together, these are considered counter-regulatory hormones — they combat insulin's blood-sugar-lowering effects, ensuring they raise blood sugar.

Such natural spikes of circadian hormones ready our bodies for the day ahead. We're never quite as relaxed as when we're in a deep sleep after all. These hormones therefore gently get us ready to wake up. Glucagon tells the liver to start squeezing glucose out. Adrenaline brings the vitality into our bodies. Growth hormone is active in cell regeneration, and new protein synthesis. The stress hormone, cortisol, grows as a general activator. These hormones all peak in the early hours of the morning and then fall to low levels during the day.

Since these chemicals all appear to increase blood sugar as part of planning for the next day, we would expect our blood sugar to fly through the roof early in the morning. This usually doesn't happen. Why? Insulin also increases early in the morning to ensure blood sugar isn't going too high.

Thus even in non-diabetics, blood sugar is not stable throughout the circadian cycle of twenty-four hours. It is just that in non-diabetics, the early morning increase in blood sugar is very low, so it's easily missed.

Yet insulin has trouble placing the brakes on people with insulin resistance— the body doesn't respond to its warnings. Because the counter-regulatory hormones are still functioning, unopposed blood sugar increases, leading to higher than normal blood sugar early in the morning.

The same pattern is seen at every time of day during the fasting. During fasting the hormonal changes include rises in growth hormone, adrenaline, glucagon, and cortisol— the same hormonal mixture produced until awakening. As you go high, the insulin decreases, but these hormones also induce the release of released sugar into the bloodstream, which raises blood sugar levels.

Insulin transfers the insulin from the blood to the tissues (liver), where it cannot be detected. It's like moving your garbage from the kitchen to under your bed. It looks like it does, but you can't see it. When the levels of insulin drop, that garbage starts moving back into the kitchen and we see higher blood sugar.

Is this morning glucose rise, or something worrisome during extended fasting? Yes, definitely not. Think about it this way: if you fasted for two days and found high sugar in the blood, where did the sugar come from? It could have just come from your own blood, the liver in particular. The glucose molecule has always been in your blood, but now you're concerned, because you can see it.

The Dawn Phenomenon, in which you see increased blood sugar during fasting, does not mean that you are doing anything wrong. It's just a normal happening. It just means you have to do more work to clear out the sugar stored. Yet, with time, that's going to do fasting.

What changed in the last fifty years or so is that we held all the celebrations but cut all the fast. The natural balance was broken and the predictable result is obesity. If you're feasting, you've got to fast. That is all there really is to it.

But if obesity is the product of eating failure, what happens if you lose all of the feasting? Well, life's getting a bit less special. If you are the guy at the wedding who is not going to drink, you are not going to eat the cake, you are not going to eat the full meal, you are not going to eat the appetizers— there is a term for that: the party pooper. And nobody wants to be the pooper in the crowd.

Eating Out

Socializing around meals plays an important part of our lives. We also get together for a dinner or a coffee with colleagues. This is common, ordinary and a part of the worldwide human culture. It's clearly not a winning strategy to try to fight that. Avoiding all social situations while fasting is not safe, and is likely to result in long-term failure to comply.

Adapt fasting into your routine, not the reverse. If you know you will have a big dinner, then skip breakfast and lunch. One of the easiest ways to incorporate fasting into your life is to skip breakfast, as it's not a meal that we socialize like lunch or dinner. It's easy to skipping breakfast during working days without anyone noticing. This will allow you to quick for sixteen hours, quite easily.

Lunch is also fairly easy to miss on the workdays: actually work through lunch. This allows you to slip fast without any special effort in a 24-hour time. Other benefits are added, too. You can get more work done, so maybe you can leave earlier. You might forget to be hungry, because you're keeping busy. Save some gas, too. And unless you go out with the same crowd to lunch every day, nobody can even notice that. Save time and money by getting thinner? Not really a bad deal.

Frequently Asked Questions

•Will fasting make me confused or forgetful?

No. During your fast you should not feel any loss in memory or focus. Fasting, on the contrary, improves both mental clarity and acuity. Fasting can in turn help to improve memory over the long term. One hypothesis is that fasting stimulates a type of cellular cleaning called autophagy, which can help prevent memory loss associated with aging.

•Does fasting lead to overeating?

The simple answer is yes, right after fasting you'll be eating more than normal. Nevertheless, the amount of food eaten on non-fasting days above the baseline is not adequate to balance the previous fast. A thirty-six-hour fasts study shows that the meal eaten after the fast is almost 20 per cent larger than usual, but there was still a net deficit of 1,958 calories over the whole two-day duration. The "overeaten" sum did not quite make up for the high. The study concludes, "A quick 36-hour did not induce a strong, unconditional stimulus to counteract the following day.

•My stomach is always growling. What can I do?

Try to drink some tea. The mechanism remains uncertain but some of the minerals are thought to help settle the stomach.

- •I take medications with food. What can I do during fasting?

Many medications may induce side effects on an empty stomach: Aspirin can cause stomach upset or ulcers. Iron supplements can cause vomiting and nausea. Metformin, which is often used for diabetes, may cause diarrhea or nausea. Talk to your doctor about whether or not these medications need to be continued during your fast time. You can also try to take your medicine with a small portion of leafy greens that is low in calories and may not interfere with your speed.

Occasionally, blood pressure can decrease during fasting. When you take medications that lower blood pressure, you can feel your blood pressure becoming too weak, which induces lightheadedness. Talk to your doctor before changing your drugs.

What if I have diabetes?

If you have type 1 or type 2-diabetes, or are taking diabetic medicines, special care must be taken. (Certain diabetes medicines, such as metformin, are used for other conditions, such as polycystic ovarian syndrome.) Monitor your blood sugar closely and adjust your medicines accordingly. The physician is expected to monitor closely. If you can't be closely followed, don't go fast.

Fasting decreases blood sugar. Unless you continue to take the same dosage of diabetes drugs, particularly insulin, your blood sugar may become extremely low, leading to hypoglycemia, during your fast. That can be a condition that is life-threatening. To lift your blood sugar back to normal, you have to take some sugar or water, even if that means you have to stop your fast for that day. During your fast you have to control your blood sugar closely. If you have low blood sugar regularly, that means that you are over-medicated and not that the method of fasting is not effective.

Can I exercise while fasting?

Most people assume that while fasting it will be impossible to exercise and sometimes those with physically demanding jobs fear about fasting while working.

Yes, exercising requires extra body power. The method of using stored food energy in a fast nevertheless remains the same. The body begins by burning glycogen, the sugar that's stored in the liver. Because there is extra energy pressure during exercise, glycogen wears out faster than it does otherwise. Yet the body usually holds twenty-four hours of ample glycogen, so it can handle a reasonable amount of exercise before it runs out.

A Day In The Life Of Intermittent Fasting

It would be near impossible to give a guideline on how to live your life because there are different intermittent fasting plans. Regardless of this, there are a few tips which might help you adhere to your intermittent fasting plan.

1. Know your goals: You need to understand the intermittent fasting plan you want and know your calorie numbers. You need to know how many calories you need to consume and how many to burn. In the event you are trying to build your body, you will need a calorie surplus. This means you will be consuming all your calories during your feeding period. With this system, you are unlikely to gain fat.

2. Know your schedule: In as much as you are focusing on the food, you eat, you also need to focus on the timing. The feeding and fasting periods are the key to intermittent fasting. People tend to check their schedule for timing and planning constantly, and all this can be avoided with proper planning. Go through your schedule and preferences. What time do you wake up from sleep? What time is your lunch break? Do you prefer to eat breakfast or dinner/supper? It is

imperative to know your preferences and schedule, as this helps you chose the best intermittent fasting plan.

3.Working out: It is important that embark on an exercise program that won't put a strain on your body. You need to know the time you will be training and whether you will be training on an empty stomach. It is imperative to eat after workouts as this helps your body get the desired fuel it needs to increase your metabolic rate.

Conclusion

And as you've seen in this book from all of the experience, intermittent fasting will help you to live better and fight diseases as you age.

There are many different diets to choose from, and whatever time of day you're busy, you should match the fasting in to suit yourself.

There will be moments when you find it difficult and when you want to give up there will be times, and this is the safest time to seek guidance from others who have been through the same thing.